Join our mailing list to be notified of new products!

www.scholasticartepress.com

Copyright © 2022 by Scholastic Arte Press All rights reserved. This book or any portion thereof may not be reproduced or used in any manner whatsoever without the express written permission of the publisher except for the use of brief quotations in a book review. Printed in the United States of America First Printing, 2022 Scholastic Arte Press www.scholasticartepress.com

Table Of Contents

Introduction 1
    Basics of Strength Training, Its Importance, and Considerations for Seniors........ 1

Benefits of Senior Strength Training..7
    Exploring how strength training can improve the quality of life for seniors.......... 7

The Vital Role of Medical Clearance and Professional Guidance...........13

Building Bone Health Through Strength Training................................19

Mind-Body Benefits of Strength Training for Seniors 26
    Exploring the mental health and cognitive benefits of engaging in regular strength training.. 26

Nutrition & Hydration for Muscle Health..33

Importance of Staying Hydrated 40

Easing Joint Pain Through Strength Training..46
    Exploring How Properly Designed Strength Training Routines Can Alleviate Joint Discomfort... 46

Choosing the Right Exercises 52
    Low-impact and Joint-Friendly Exercises Suitable for Seniors 52

Progressive Overload and Adaptation 58

Balancing Cardiovascular and Strength Training....................................65

Tracking Progress and Staying Motivated 72
    Setting realistic goals and measuring achievements... 72

Mindful Ageing Through Strength Training..79
    Exploring the concept of aging mindfully and how strength training can support it 79

Senior Success Stories in Strength Training 86
Sharing real-life stories of seniors who have benefited from incorporating strength training into their lives 86
Illustrated Guide of Strength and Balance Exercises for Seniors 91

Introduction

Basics of Strength Training, Its Importance, and Considerations for Seniors

---

Buckle up because we're about to explore a fascinating topic that could redefine how we spend our golden years - Senior Strength Training. Elegantly maturing folks, radiating vitality, self-assurance, and a real passion for living. What's their secret, you ask? It's the power of strength training tailored specifically for seniors.

The Power of Strength Training for Seniors

It's no big secret that as we get older, our bodies start to go through some changes. We might notice our muscles getting a bit smaller, our bones not feeling as strong, and maybe our overall power taking a bit of a hit. But seriously, don't let that get you down. Here comes something cool: strength training. And guess what? It's not only for the young and full of energy. Seniors can totally get in on this action too.

Being able to pick up your groceries without even thinking about it, having a blast playing with your grandkids, or finally going on those awesome adventures you've always dreamed about. That's where strength training swoops in. Not only does strength training help you keep and build your muscles, but it's also a superstar for your bones. Muscles and bones can work together like an epic dance routine, giving you balance and lowering the chances of taking a tumble. And get this: the benefits aren't just physical. Strength training is like a mood booster, a brain sharpener, and an overall life enhancer.

Why Senior Strength?

Now, you might be thinking, "Why senior-specific strength training? Can't I just follow any old workout routine?" Great question! Senior strength training isn't about trying to keep up with the younger crowd. That's why senior strength training focuses on a few key principles:

1. Safety First: You know, when we're talking about our own bodies, making sure we're safe should always be at the forefront of our minds, don't you think? A senior-oriented program takes into account any existing health conditions or limitations you might have. This ensures that you exercise safely and effectively. It considers any health issues you might be dealing with, such as a tricky knee or a wonky back. By customizing the exercises to fit your specific situation, you're making sure you build strength without jeopardizing your well-being. Similar to how you wouldn't plunge into the deep end of a pool without strong swimming skills, it's wise to avoid leaping into demanding workouts that your body might not be fully prepared for.

2. Progressive Approach: The key isn't to immediately tackle the heaviest weights head-on. For those of us who've been around a bit, when we embark on a senior-focused strength training regimen, we usually kick off with weights that are quite manageable. The idea is to allow our body to become familiar with the heightened demand. It's akin to how we wouldn't even dream of running a marathon without some serious training beforehand. Similarly, aiming to lift weights like a seasoned bodybuilder requires a step-by-step progression. This methodical approach does wonders for our muscles and bones, facilitating their adaptation and gradual strengthening, all without the sensation of trying to lift a mountain.

3. Flexibility and Mobility: Many of these programs tend to blend in stretches and exercises that do wonders for your flexibility and how smoothly you can move around. It's pretty crucial since it helps your joints keep up their full range of motion. The senior strength training is well thought-out to make sure those stretches and motions are there, so your joints stay limber and your body keeps its fluid motion.

4. Social Engagement: Many senior strength training classes foster a sense of community. Working out with people who share your vibe can really amp up the whole fitness adventure. There are these cool programs that set you up in classes where it's not just about the exercise grind, but you're sweating it out with folks who are sailing in the same boat. Imagine having your own personal cheer squad, egging you on, and turning the whole sweaty affair into a blast! Just like everything's better with friends, workouts included!

That being said, strength training can also help with the following issues

1. **Empowering Bones and Beating Osteoporosis**

   Osteoporosis, often referred to as the "silent disease," weakens bones and makes them susceptible to fractures. For seniors, it's a significant concern that can limit mobility and independence. When you do these exercises that put a bit of pressure on your bones, it's like giving them a little nudge to grow. They become denser and tougher. So, stuff like squats, lunges, and even those elastic band thingamajigs can do wonders to keep your bones super solid.

2. **Finding Equilibrium and Defying Balance Issues**

   Maintaining balance becomes trickier as we age, leading to falls that can have severe consequences. Senior strength training comes to the rescue again, as it targets the muscles responsible for stability. The strengthening of core muscles, along with exercises like leg lifts and calf raises, can drastically improve balance. This not only prevents falls but also instills a sense of confidence and assurance in daily activities.

3. **Battling Obesity through Muscle Building**

   Obesity is a pressing concern among seniors that can exacerbate other health issues. Strength training for older adults, when combined with a well-rounded eating plan, emerges as quite the formidable ally in the battle against obesity. While aerobic activities torch those calories while you're in motion, activities that help build those muscles maintain that higher calorie-burning state even after you've wrapped up your exercise session. So, by weaving strength training into your regular routine, you're pretty much giving your body a nudge to become this amazing calorie-burning engine.

4. **Boosting Joint Health**

   Arthritis, with its persistent joint pain, can hinder the enjoyment of life. However, contrary to common belief, physical activity can be incredibly beneficial for arthritis sufferers. Senior strength training, when executed under proper guidance, can actually alleviate arthritis symptoms. It helps in maintaining joint flexibility and range of motion, reduces pain through improved muscular support around the joints, and boosts the production of synovial fluid, which lubricates the joints. Low-impact exercises like swimming, resistance band stretches, and seated leg lifts are excellent choices for seniors with arthritis.

5. **Bid Adieu to Back Problems**

   Back problems are a common woe among the elderly, often stemming from weakened back muscles and poor posture. Senior strength training comes into play here too, by targeting the muscles of the back and the core. Exercises like bridges, supermans, and seated rows can help strengthen the muscles that support the spine, alleviating back pain and improving overall posture.

Strength Training Exercises for Senior

Bird Dog: Balancing Gracefully

A beautiful fusion of balance and strength, it engages both your core and back muscles. Begin on all fours, and extend your right arm forward while simultaneously lifting your left leg behind you. Hold for a brief moment, feeling the gentle contraction in your abdominal muscles. Then, switch sides. This exercise not only enhances stability but also supports a healthy spine.

Eccentric Straight Leg Raise: Defying Gravity Safely

The Eccentric Straight Leg Raise is a splendid way to bolster the muscles surrounding your hips and thighs. To do this work out, just lay on your back. Bend one leg and have the other leg pointing straight up into the air. Slowly lower the raised leg towards the ground, taking about four to five seconds. This controlled motion engages your quadriceps and promotes joint flexibility, helping you to tackle daily movements with ease.

Cat and Camel: Embracing Spinal Serenity

Imagine a cat arching its back in the most luxurious stretch – that's the inspiration behind the Cat and Camel exercise. This fluid movement releases tension along your spine, offering a soothing experience. While on all fours, arch your back towards the ceiling as you inhale, resembling the "camel" pose. Then, round your back towards the floor as you exhale, akin to the stretch a cat performs. This exercise nurtures your spinal flexibility and helps maintain good posture.

Leg Extensions: Empowering Mobility

Simple yet impactful, leg extensions are a fantastic way to enhance lower body strength. Find a sturdy chair and sit comfortably. Begin by extending one leg straight out in front of you, holding it for a moment before lowering it down. This exercise targets your quadriceps while promoting knee stability. As you gracefully extend your leg, you're also extending your ability to relish life's many experiences.

Glute Bridge: Building Bridges to Stamina

First, find a comfy spot to lie down on your back. Go ahead and bend those knees of yours, and plant your feet nice and flat on the floor. Gently lift up your hips off the ground. Just envision creating this nice straight line from your shoulders all the way down to your knees. Oh, and don't forget about those glutes (you know, your backside muscles)! Then, slowly lower your hips back down. Give it a shot and feel the burn in all the right places! This exercise not only invigorates your posterior chain but also helps combat lower back discomfort.

Kneeling Shoulder Tap Push-Up: A Test of Balance and Strength

Our first stop on this fitness journey takes us to the dynamic Kneeling Shoulder Tap Push-Up. This exercise not only works those upper body muscles but also challenges our balance and core stability. Start in a plank position on your knees, keeping your body in a straight line from head to knees. Engage your core and maintain stability as you lift one hand to tap the opposite shoulder. Feel the burn in your arms and core as you alternate sides. This exercise is perfect for building functional strength and boosting confidence in your body's abilities.

Hip Flexion: Embrace Flexibility and Range of Motion

Next up, we're delving into hip flexion exercises. These movements are all about maintaining flexibility and range of motion in the hips, a crucial aspect of senior strength training. One simple yet effective exercise involves lying on your back and gently bringing one knee towards your chest. Hold the stretch for a few seconds, then switch sides. Feel those hips saying "thank you" as you give them the attention they deserve.

Shifting Weight: A Fun Dance of Strength

Ah, the beauty of shifting weight exercises – they're like a dance routine for your muscles. Start by standing tall and slowly shifting your weight from one foot to the other. Imagine you're swaying to your favorite tune while building strength in your legs and core. You can even spice it up by holding onto a sturdy surface with one hand, challenging your balance and stability. It's like a two-in-one workout: physical strength and a dance party!

Resistance Band Workouts: Your Portable Gym

Now, let's talk about the fantastic world of resistance band workouts. These flexible, colorful bands are like your own portable gym. Attach one to a secure surface and engage in exercises like bicep curls, chest presses, and seated rows. They provide gentle resistance that's easy on the joints but still effective in building strength. The best part? You can take these bands anywhere – perfect for those who love to stay active while on the go.

Calf Raises: Rising to the Occasion

Our final stop in this senior strength training journey takes us to calf raises. These easy-peasy moves focus on those calf muscles – you know, the ones that are all about keeping you steady and balanced? So, put your feet sort of-hip distance away from each other, gently lift yourself onto your tippy-toes, and then gently come back down. Feel the burn as you strengthen your calves and work on preventing falls. It's a small move with big benefits!

So, there you have it – the lowdown on senior strength training and why it's an absolute game-changer for those golden years. Keep this in mind: age is truly just a number, and if you take the right approach, you can mature like a fine wine, growing more exceptional and resilient as the years go by.

Keep that curiosity alive and your spirits high! Stay strong, my friends.

Benefits of Senior Strength Training

Exploring how strength training can improve the quality of life for seniors

---

Life's journey is quite a ride, isn't it? And while we're on this adventure, one thing is for sure: we all get older. With time, we become wiser, gather stories, and start new chapters. But, as the years go by, our bodies change too. That's where senior strength training steps in - it's like our secret weapon to help us keep that youthful spark as we age.

What is Strength Training?

Lifting weights, often referred to as strength training or resistance workouts, involves performing specific exercises that target particular muscle sets by introducing resistance or added weight. You know, there's something about those workouts that really make your heart race – they're fantastic for giving your endurance a real boost! But let's chat about strength training for a second. The whole idea here is to up your physical strength game and just make everyday movements feel smoother. The key to making strength training seriously effective is to gently nudge those muscles to do a little more each time you hit the gym. And guess what? You can pull this off with some trusty dumbbells, stretchy resistance bands, or just your own body weight. Pretty awesome, right?

Building Healthier Bodies as We Age

The aging process is natural and beautiful, but it does come with a few downsides, such as decreased muscle mass, bone density, and joint flexibility. This is where the magic of senior strength training steps in. Through consistently doing strength training, you can truly achieve great benefits for your overall well-being, both internally and externally.

Benefits:

Here are some of the benefits that you can get by regularly adding strength training to your life:

1. Increases Your Ability to Perform Activities of Daily Living (ADLs)

A life where you can effortlessly carry your groceries, walk up the stairs without feeling winded, and maintain your independence in day-to-day tasks. That's the gift senior strength training bestows upon us. As we age, the ability to perform ADLs becomes crucial for maintaining our quality of life. Strength training targets the muscle groups necessary for these activities, making them not only achievable but also enjoyable. From picking up grandchildren to tending to our gardens, strength training ensures we continue to relish life's simple pleasures.

2. Reduces Your Chances of Falling

As we grow older, one thing that often worries us is the possibility of taking a tumble. These falls can result in pretty serious injuries, affecting not only our physical health but also how we feel inside. However, strength training acts as a reliable armor against this threat. By enhancing muscle strength and balance, seniors can significantly reduce their chances of taking a tumble. A substantial body and improved balance mean that even uneven terrains or unexpected obstacles are less likely to catch us off guard. With a stable foundation, we can confidently step into each day, knowing that we're equipped to navigate the world safely.

3. Guarding Against Illness

As we journey through life, our immune system sometimes needs an extra boost to fend off various illnesses that might come knocking. Participating in consistent strength training as we age has been found to have a positive impact on our immune system. This translates to fewer instances of falling sick and more opportunities to relish in the joys of life. Of course, I'm not suggesting you'll become invincible against all colds, but having that added layer of defense surely sounds appealing, doesn't it?

4. Maintaining Strong Bones

Bones – the framework that supports us throughout our lives. One of the unsung heroes of senior strength training is its positive impact on bone health. By engaging in weight-bearing exercises, you're giving your bones a reason to stay strong and resilient. This could actually be pretty helpful in guarding against fractures, which tend to sneak up more as we get older. It's like giving your bones some bonus protection for all the exciting stuff coming our way!

5. The Muscle Revival

You might be familiar with the old saying, "If you don't use it, you lose it," Well, it's pretty interesting how that applies to our muscle mass. As we get older, our muscles kind of shrink, and that can lead to a decrease in how strong we are and how easily we can move around. Senior strength training comes to the rescue. By incorporating resistance exercises into your routine, you're essentially telling your muscles that they're still needed and valued. This can result in increased muscle mass and improved functional abilities – think of it as a personal invitation to reclaim your youthful energy.

6. Revitalizing Functional Movement

The feeling of moving freely and effortlessly – something we often take for granted. But as we age, maintaining functional movement becomes paramount. That's where senior strength training comes to the rescue! Engaging in regular resistance exercises not only strengthens muscles but also enhances joint flexibility and stability. Imagine being able to pick up your grandkids without a second thought or enjoying a leisurely stroll without those pesky aches. Senior strength training can turn these dreams into reality, making everyday activities a breeze.

7. A Better Body Composition

Let's be honest, who doesn't want to look and feel their best, regardless of age? Senior strength training has got your back on that one too. As we grow older, our metabolism might decide to slow down a bit, and unwanted flab might become a more familiar companion. No need to stress, because diving into weightlifting can actually be quite advantageous. When you dedicate yourself to building those sleek muscles, your metabolism receives a nice little push. This means your body becomes a pro at torching calories, working like a champ even when you're not pumping iron. So, it's not just about the iron-pumping sessions! Plus, with improved muscle tone, you'll find that your posture gets a boost, making you stand tall and proud.

8. Efficiency in calorie-burning

Now, let's talk about everyone's favorite topic – burning calories! Senior strength training is like adding a turbocharger to your metabolism engine. Those muscles you're building through resistance exercises demand more energy, which means your body becomes a calorie-burning machine, even at rest. It's like getting a gold star for your efforts – you not only sculpt your physique but also keep that sneaky weight gain at bay.

Mental Well-being:

Strength training for older adults goes beyond merely enhancing muscle mass and bone strength; it's a real transformative adventure that perks up the mind just as it does the body. Science has confirmed time and again that when you get moving, your body unleashes those delightful endorphins, the natural mood boosters.

1. Lower Risk of Dementia and Alzheimer's

The link between senior strength training and keeping a sharp mind is truly intriguing. Research has shown that when you engage in strength training, it can actually prompt your body to produce a specific protein called brain-derived neurotrophic factor (BDNF). This unique protein has a crucial job in looking after your brain's well-being. It encourages the growth of fresh neurons and synapses, which essentially helps lower the chances of dealing with memory decline, dementia, and even Alzheimer's disease. By taking on exercises that challenge both the body and the brain, older adults can genuinely strive to keep their mental sharpness intact as they enjoy their later years in life.

2. Increased Happiness

You know, there's something pretty cool that happens when we share a good laugh – it totally boosts our mood. But get this, ever heard that hitting the gym for some strength training can do the same? Yep, turns out that when we get moving and lifting, our bodies let out these awesome chemicals called endorphins. They're like our very own natural mood lifters. They not only help us deal with pain but also make us feel super happy and, you guessed it, euphoric. So, if you're a senior looking to fight off those blues, regular sessions of strength training could be like your personal happiness fountain. It's like waving goodbye to feeling down and lonely and saying hello to a brighter emotional state.

3. Boosts Your Self-esteem

Aging often comes with its share of challenges, and maintaining a positive self-image can become increasingly difficult. This is where senior strength training shines as a beacon of empowerment. As seniors witness their physical strength and endurance improve, a profound shift occurs in their perception of self. The sense of accomplishment that comes from setting fitness goals and achieving them can significantly boost self-esteem and self-worth. With each successful lift and every milestone reached, seniors reaffirm their capabilities and unlock a renewed sense of confidence.

FAQs Regarding Senior Strength Training:

1. Isn't Strength Training for the Younger Generation?

Absolutely not! While strength training is often associated with younger individuals, it's equally essential for seniors. As we age, our muscles naturally weaken, making daily activities more challenging. Strength training helps counteract this muscle loss, making everyday tasks easier and enhancing your quality of life.

2. Will Strength Training Make Me Bulky?

Don't sweat it at all! It's all about building up sleek muscle and giving your bones a boost in density. The goal is improved functional strength and overall health, not bodybuilding.

3. Can Strength Training Improve My Balance and Coordination?

Definitely! Balance and coordination tend to decline with age, leading to an increased risk of falls. Strength training targets the muscles that support balance, helping you maintain stability and reducing the likelihood of accidents.

4. Will Strength Training Help with Arthritis?

Yes, it can! Gentle strength training exercises can help alleviate arthritis symptoms by increasing joint flexibility and reducing pain. Always consult a professional to tailor exercises to your specific needs.

5. Can Strength Training Boost My Metabolism?

Absolutely. Muscle burns more calories at rest than fat does, so increasing your muscle mass through strength training can give your metabolism a boost, helping with weight management.

6. Is Strength Training Safe for Someone with Existing Health Conditions?

Yes, in many cases, but here's the thing– it's really crucial to discuss with your doctor before you jump headfirst into any fresh exercise plan, especially if you've got other health bits to consider. A professional can guide you on which exercises won't stir up problems and might even lend a hand with your specific condition.

7. Can Strength Training Improve My Mood and Mental Health?

Definitely. Participating in physical activities like strength training has this amazing way of releasing endorphins, those natural mood boosters our body loves. When we make a habit of fitting in those strength training sessions often, it's like giving stress, anxiety, and gloomy feelings a run for their money.

Getting Started – Your Personal Journey

Before you dive into your exciting journey of senior strength training, it's really important to keep in mind that seeking advice from a healthcare expert is a smart move, especially if you have any existing health concerns. Once you've got the green signal, think about kicking off with a certified personal trainer who's all about senior fitness. They really excel at making a personalized plan that fits you like a glove and ensuring you're on the mark with every step, leaving no room for any slip-ups.

In our rapidly evolving world filled with amazing technological advancements and trendy innovations, there are certain aspects that remain constant. One such unchanging truth is the immense importance of maintaining good health and vitality as we journey through the process of aging. And that's where senior strength training steps in. It hands us the means we need to live awesome lives even when we're way past our prime. By getting into the whole strength training thing, we're basically investing in a future that's all about energy, freedom, and making the most of every second. So, why not grab those weights, get those resistance bands out, and start this journey toward a brighter, stronger tomorrow?

The Vital Role of Medical Clearance and Professional Guidance

In a world brimming with information, where the internet generously serves up a wealth of health-related guidance and self-help tips, it's tempting to believe we can tackle our medical issues all by ourselves. But there's a crucial facet of healthcare that often slips through the cracks as we hunt for speedy fixes: seeking professional medical clearance and guidance. In this piece, we're going to explore precisely what medical clearance involves and underscore the critical role it plays in safeguarding our well-being.

What is Medical Clearance?

Medical clearance, in essence, represents a formal evaluation carried out by seasoned medical experts. This thorough assessment aims to gauge an individual's holistic state of health and make informed judgments about their appropriateness for particular activities or medical procedures. It acts as a comprehensive examination, essentially verifying that an individual possesses the physical and mental fitness necessary to participate in an array of endeavors, spanning from travel to surgical procedures, and everything encompassed therein.

The Importance of Medical Clearance

Comprehensive medical clearance serves as a vital cornerstone of healthcare practice. Prior to executing any medical operation, it includes a comprehensive examination and research of a patient's overall health. This assessment takes into account a variety of criteria, including the patient's medical history, any pre-existing medical issues, allergies, and current prescription regimen. It also considers the patient's emotional and mental well-being, recognizing the substantial influence it may have on their physical health.

This thorough medical examination offers healthcare practitioners with a full picture of their patient's health. As a consequence, they can devise treatment plans that are both effective and safe. This method detects any possible difficulties or contraindications, ensuring that medical procedures and treatments do not harm the patient accidentally.

Here are a few reasons why you should obtain Medical Clearance:

1. Safety First

One of the primary motivations behind obtaining medical clearance is ensuring safety. When you consult with healthcare experts, they carefully evaluate your health status, current medications, and medical background. Their aim is to pinpoint any possible hazards related to your intended pursuits. Whether you're contemplating activities like scuba diving, preparing for surgery, or embarking on a fresh exercise routine, seeking medical clearance is a precautionary measure to guarantee that your well-being remains uncompromised.

2. Personalized Health Guidance

Each of us is unique, and our health needs vary accordingly. Seeking medical clearance allows you to receive personalized guidance from healthcare experts who understand your individual circumstances. This tailored advice can make a significant difference in managing chronic conditions, preventing potential health issues, or optimizing your overall well-being.

3. Legal and Ethical Responsibility

In many situations, obtaining medical clearance is not just advisable but a legal and ethical requirement. Medical professionals must ensure that patients are fit to undergo certain medical procedures, participate in sports, or engage in potentially risky activities. This not only protects the individual but also safeguards healthcare providers from potential legal consequences.

4. Early Detection and Prevention

Medical clearance often involves a series of tests and assessments that can detect underlying health issues even before symptoms become apparent. By identifying these issues early, medical professionals can recommend interventions or lifestyle changes that can prevent more severe health problems down the road.

5. Peace of Mind

Receiving the green light from a certified healthcare professional can be incredibly comforting. Having that expert validation that your health choices are on the right path, be it for a significant life change or merely pursuing a healthier lifestyle, can offer you a genuine sense of reassurance.

6. Professional Expertise

Medical specialists with years of rigorous study and practical experience have the competence required to provide accurate and dependable counsel. Relying solely on self-diagnosis or internet advice can be risky and lead to unnecessary anxiety.

What Can I Expect at the Medical Clearance Exam?

Recognizing the importance of obtaining medical clearance naturally prompts the question: What exactly does a medical clearance examination entail? This inquiry is quite valid, especially for individuals who might not be well-versed in the process.

A medical clearance examination is essentially a thorough evaluation of a patient's overall health. It includes a thorough study of the patient's medical history, a physical examination, and, on occasion, the addition of specific tests or consultations with other medical professionals. Here's a more detailed explanation of what this entails:

Delving into Medical History: The process kicks off with a meticulous examination of the patient's medical background. This encompasses chronic conditions, past surgical procedures, allergies, and the medications presently in use. It's vital to divulge all relevant details, as any omissions could result in an incomplete assessment.

The Medical Assessment: When you step into a healthcare setting, your journey towards better health often begins with a comprehensive physical examination. This check-up is a crucial step to evaluate your overall well-being. During this process, healthcare professionals carefully monitor vital signs like blood pressure, heart rate, and respiration rate. Additionally, they delve deeper, conducting a thorough examination of your heart and lungs to detect any signs of infection and gauge your general physical condition.

Exploring through Labs: Depending on your medical history and the nature of your upcoming treatment, laboratory investigations may be deemed necessary. These investigations encompass a range of tests, from basic blood work to more specialized assessments like electrocardiograms and various imaging techniques such as X-rays or ultrasounds. These tests serve the vital purpose of providing a more comprehensive understanding of your overall health.

Seeking Expert Insights: In certain situations, your primary physician may opt for a collaborative approach. This involves consulting with specialists to ensure that the planned procedure is suitable for your unique health circumstances. For instance, if you have a history of heart-related issues, your doctor might seek the expertise of a cardiologist, who can offer valuable insights into the condition of your heart.

A medical clearance test is essentially a rigorous process aimed to guarantee that a patient is in the best possible condition to safely undertake a medical operation. It leaves no stone untouched, including a thorough assessment of medical history, a complete physical examination, and the appropriate utilization of laboratory testing and specialist consultations. This method is intended to protect the patient's well-being and provide a smooth medical journey.

Addressing Risk Factors

One of the fundamental aspects of prioritizing health is recognizing and managing risk factors. Think of risk factors as pieces of the health puzzle unique to each of us. These factors can stem from our lifestyle choices or even our genetic blueprint, influencing our susceptibility to various health conditions. They run the gamut from what we eat and how active we are to the health history written in our family tree. Understanding and tending to these risk factors is like securing the foundation of our well-being.

Someone who comes from a family with a long history of heart disease. This person's daily routine mostly consists of lounging on the couch and indulging in a diet loaded with artery-clogging saturated fats. They might not realize the storm of risks brewing within them if they don't seek expert guidance. Yet, with the wisdom of a healthcare professional, they gain a clearer view of their health risk landscape. Armed with this knowledge, they can proactively embrace changes like tweaking their eating habits and embracing a regular exercise regimen, all tailored to curbing those lurking risks.

Moreover, risk factors can sometimes be hidden or subtle. Conditions like hypertension or high cholesterol often manifest without noticeable symptoms. A yearly check-up with a healthcare practitioner can help in early identification and action. This preventative strategy has the potential to significantly improve people's long-term health results.

The Role of Professional Guidance

In the intricate realm of healthcare, the significance of professional guidance cannot be emphasized enough. Medical experts, armed with extensive years of education and hands-on experience, stand as the stalwarts safeguarding the well-being of patients. Their knowledge is the compass guiding critical decisions concerning diagnosis, treatment, and the overall care of individuals.

The scope of professional guidance extends beyond the confines of clinical walls; it encompasses ethical and legal dimensions as well. Healthcare practitioners have a thorough awareness of the legal and ethical frameworks that govern their profession. They are skilled at navigating the maze of rules, ensuring that all actions comply with ethical ideals and are within the confines of the law.

Furthermore, healthcare workers excel in guiding patients to make well-informed healthcare decisions. This encompasses discussions on various treatment avenues, lifestyle adjustments, and preventive measures. The presence of a trusted medical advisor can significantly bolster an individual's confidence in dealing with health-related matters.

In intricate medical scenarios, such as chronic ailments or severe injuries, healthcare professionals assume an irreplaceable role in orchestrating care, tracking progress, and adapting treatment plans as necessary. Their expertise guarantees that individuals receive the most effective and secure interventions available.

A Symbiotic Relationship

Medical clearance and professional guidance share a symbiotic relationship. They work hand in hand to safeguard both patients and healthcare providers. A thorough medical clearance equips professionals with the vital data they need to make well-informed decisions, effectively lowering the chances of facing malpractice claims. In parallel, expert advice guarantees that these decisions not only align with medical best practices but also adhere to ethical and legal standards.

In Conclusion

Medical clearance should never be ignored as a necessity; it is an essential safeguard for our health and safety. Whether you're starting a new fitness journey, planning a major medical operation, or going through a major life transition, reaching out to a healthcare professional for proper medical evaluation is a choice that can genuinely improve your overall health and quality of life. Always remember that your health is an asset too valuable to jeopardize; receiving advice from a skilled professional is the surefire method to ensure you're on the correct track.

Building Bone Health Through Strength Training

When we're thinking about keeping ourselves in good shape, we tend to put a lot of attention on things like staying in good physical condition and keeping up our strength. But you know, it's easy to overlook the importance of taking care of our bones in the midst of all that. It's kind of like how we put effort into building up our muscles, our bones need some TLC too to stay tough and dense. So, let's have a little chat about how staying active, especially when we do strength training, plays a pretty cool role in looking after the health of our bones. We'll delve into how such training plays a pivotal role in preventing bone loss and promoting skeletal wellness.

Exercise and Bone Density: A Symbiotic Connection

When we think about exercise, we often envision toned muscles and improved cardiovascular health. However, our bones also reap substantial benefits from physical activity. Engaging in activities that put weight on your bones, like walking, running, and dancing, has been linked to making your bones stronger for quite a while. But what about strength training?

In recent years, research has illuminated the profound impact of strength training on bone health. The process isn't solely about building muscle; it involves stimulating bone tissue to adapt and become more resilient. Weightlifting, bodyweight exercises, and resistance band workouts engage the bones in ways that encourage the deposition of minerals like calcium, making them denser and less prone to fractures.

How effective is resistance training in promoting bone health?

Have you ever pondered whether those weightlifting sessions contribute significantly to your bone well-being? The answer comes back loud and clear—absolutely! Resistance training, often anointed as strength training, encompasses tasks such as lifting weights, harnessing resistance bands, or even utilizing your own body weight to generate resistance. This workout style exerts a certain pressure on your bones, consequently activating your body's natural bone-enhancing mechanism.

As you partake in resistance training, your bones undergo a transformative process, rendering them denser and more robust. The mechanical stress from lifting weights encourages bone-forming cells to kick into high gear, leading to increased bone mineral density. Now, don't worry if these terms sound a bit scientific – all you need to know is that stronger bones mean better protection against fractures and osteoporosis down the line.

How Does Resistance Training Prevent Bone Loss?

1. Mechanical Stress: One of the primary mechanisms through which resistance training bolsters bone health is by subjecting bones to mechanical stress. When we do weightlift, all that pulling and pushing we do with the weights? It puts some stress on our bones. Our bones actually get stronger because they're trying to handle all that weight. And It's those little cells called osteoblasts. They're the ones in charge of building up new bone stuff.

2. Hormonal Influence: When you engage in resistance training, your body decides to release growth factors and hormones. These hormones, like the insulin-like growth factor (IGF-1) and testosterone, are like the VIPs of your body's growth. And They're actually helping out with bone remodeling. As bones are subjected to the stress of resistance exercises, the hormonal response enhances bone-building activity.

3. Enhanced Mineralization: Bone health isn't just about size; it's also about quality. Resistance training improves bone mineralization, ensuring that bones are fortified with essential minerals, especially calcium. This fortification enhances bone density, making them more resistant to fractures and injuries.

4. Balance and Coordination: Functional movements performed during resistance training sessions also contribute to better balance and coordination. This aspect is often overlooked but is crucial for preventing falls, especially in older adults who are more susceptible to fractures.

The Impact of Osteoporosis on Bones

Let's take a moment to reflect on the potential outcomes of not giving our bones the attention they deserve. Osteoporosis, a condition in which bones lose density and become more fragile, can have some serious downsides. Remember, osteoporosis doesn't just happen suddenly. It's a gradual process, but the lasting effects can be quite substantial. Fractures that result from osteoporosis, especially in the hip area, can really impact a person's overall life quality, their ability to remain independent, and unfortunately, even raise the chance of mortality. This really underscores the significance of looking after our bones today to prevent grappling with such challenging consequences down the road.

Are women more prone to getting osteoporosis?

The simple response would be affirmative, although there's a deeper layer to consider. Women tend to have a higher chance than men when it comes to dealing with osteoporosis. This condition makes bones more fragile and easier to break, and it seems to become even clearer when we focus on women who've gone through menopause.

During this phase, women experience a quick drop in bone density, and this is greatly affected by the decrease in estrogen levels. This situation makes women more prone to ending up with osteoporosis. Engaging in regular resistance exercises helps stimulate bone-building cells called osteoblasts. Those amazing cells do their thing by actually building up fresh bone material, which gives your bones an awesome upgrade, making them tougher and better at bouncing back.

When Should People Start Resistance Training?

When is the ideal time to begin lifting those weights, we frequently think. Well, it's never too early to start incorporating resistance training into your training regimen. Your bones expand very quickly during youth. Thus, this is the ideal moment to begin resistance training. You can use light weights and perform exercises like squats and lunges. Your bones will strengthen and expand as a result of these exercises. Including weight training in your fitness regimen can actually assist in maintaining the health of your bones, regardless of your age.

The Power of Weight Training:

When we think of weight training, we often envision muscular individuals lifting heavy weights in a gym. Weight training or you might call it strength training or resistance training, isn't just about the surface-level stuff. It's a mix of exercises all aimed at giving your muscles a real run for their money, dealing with resistance in all sorts of creative ways – think dumbbells, those stretchy resistance bands, or even just your good ol' body weight.

- **Stronger Bones and Muscles:**

    The growth of solid, well-defined muscles is the most visible benefit of weight training. A lot of people don't frequently consider how having strong bones and well-developed muscles truly go hand in hand. When we do exercises like lifting weights or putting pressure on our bodies, our muscles work on making our bones denser and tougher. This teamwork between bones and muscles is pretty amazing!

- **Bone Density:**

    Our bones tend to lose density as we get older, which increases the risk of fractures and osteoporosis. In this situation, weight training serves as a hero. The mechanical stress applied during weightlifting prompts your bones to increase their mineral density, making them less prone to fractures and overall deterioration.

- **Enhanced Balance and Posture:**

    Balance is not just about staying upright – it's about preventing falls and subsequent fractures, especially in older adults. Strength training improves your overall balance and posture by enhancing muscle coordination, reducing the risk of accidental tumbles.

- **Metabolism Boost:**

    Strength training offers benefits beyond just shaping your body – it gives your metabolism a boost as well. By developing lean muscle, your system becomes better at torching calories. This isn't just great for managing weight; it also does wonders for your bones.

- **Flexibility at Its Core:**

    What's neat about weight training is how flexible it is. You can tweak exercises to match your fitness aptitude, so whether you're a newbie or a fitness pro, it works. Whether you're into resistance bands, gym machines, or old-school free weights, you can up the challenge gradually as you get stronger.

Slowing Osteoporosis Naturally:

Osteoporosis, also known as the "silent sickness," is characterized by weakened bones that are more prone to fractures. Although it is a prevalent worry as we age, there are techniques to naturally limit its development:

- **Get Active:** Regular physical activity is like a secret weapon against osteoporosis. Engaging in weight-bearing exercises, such as walking, jogging, dancing, or even stair climbing, can help stimulate bone growth and increase bone density.

- **Avoid Smoking:** Smoking is associated with a reduction in bone density. Cigarette smoke contains chemicals that prevent the body from absorbing calcium and lower estrogen levels, both of which are vital for bone health.

- **Vitamin D & Calcium:** These two nutrients—calcium and vitamin D—are like a dynamic combo for bone health. Bones are constructed with calcium, and vitamin D aids in calcium absorption. Make sure to incorporate foods high in calcium in your diet, such as dairy products, leafy greens, and fortified items.

The maintenance of strong bones can be considerably aided by nutrient-rich diets. Include whole grains, nuts, seeds, fish, and other sources of magnesium, vitamin K, and phosphorus in your meals.

Getting Started on Weight Training for Osteoporosis

Always consult your healthcare provider before beginning any new exercise regimen. They can provide personalized advice and ensure you're taking the right approach based on your specific needs.

Now here are some osteoporosis-friendly exercises that can help strengthen bones and improve overall quality of life.

Upper Body Exercises:

Tension Without Weights: Sometimes, it's best to start simple. Engaging in gentle tension-based exercises can be incredibly effective. Think push-ups against a wall or countertop. These workouts are all about using your own body weight to help you get stronger over time, and the best part is that they're gentle on your bones so you don't have to worry about overdoing it.

Weight-Bearing Exercises: Think about going for a walk, a nice jog, or even busting a move on the dance floor. What's cool about these is that they all involve putting weight on your feet and legs, which actually helps your bones get stronger and grow over the long haul. Remember, consistency is key!

Muscle-Strengthening Exercises: Participating in some resistance-focused workouts such as those with stretchy resistance bands or opting for slightly lighter dumbbells can actually do wonders for boosting your muscle strength. Having strong muscles comes with the added perk of giving your bones more stability and cutting down on the chances of taking a tumble.

Balance Exercises: Working on your balance is essential because osteoporosis might make falling more likely. Try doing yoga or tai chi; these exercises not only improve balance but also promote mindfulness and relaxation.

Flexibility Exercises: Maintaining flexibility is often overlooked, but it plays a vital role in overall bone health. Incorporate gentle stretching into your routine to keep your muscles and joints supple.

Conclusion

While cardio workouts steal much of the fitness spotlight, the role of strength training in building and maintaining bone health is undeniable. The connection between exercise and bone density is a dynamic one, showcasing how physical activity can be a potent ally in the fight against bone loss.

Resistance training, with its unique ability to subject bones to controlled stress, hormonal influence, and enhanced mineralization, offers a comprehensive approach to preventing bone loss. Not only does it make your bones stronger, but it also boosts your overall strength, balance, and coordination.

Adding resistance training to your workout regimen is like giving your bones a friendly boost. Just like a house stands firm with a solid base, your body leans on sturdy bones to accompany you through every twist and turn in life. So, go ahead, pick up those dumbbells, flex those muscles, and set off on a mission to craft unyielding bones that will endure the trials of time.

Mind-Body Benefits of Strength Training for Seniors

Exploring the mental health and cognitive benefits of engaging in regular strength training

---

Let's dive into something that's often overlooked but holds the power to transform our golden years – strength training for seniors. As we journey through time, it becomes ever more important to maintain harmony between our mental and physical well-being. One excellent approach to accomplish this is by adopting the practice of strength training, even in our golden years. In this section, we'll explore what exactly strength training for seniors is, and more importantly, how to do it safely.

Strength Training with Safety

Safety should always be the top priority, especially for seniors diving into strength training. After all, we're aiming for improved well-being, not unnecessary risks. Now, onto the topic of safety – a crucial element when it comes to a successful strength training regimen, especially for older folks.

1. Consult Your Physician: First and foremost, you should consult with your healthcare provider before diving into any fresh fitness regimen. Doctors have the scoop on your particular health requirements and constraints, making sure you're not pushing your body too hard. They can check out your health situation and propose exercises that suit your personal necessities.

2. Qualified Trainers: These professionals understand the unique needs and limitations of older adults and can tailor a program to suit your abilities. Opt for a trainer who's well-versed in senior fitness – they understand the nuances and can

Adding resistance training to your workout regimen is like giving your bones a friendly boost. Just like a house stands firm with a solid base, your body leans on sturdy bones to accompany you through every twist and turn in life. So, go ahead, pick up those dumbbells, flex those muscles, and set off on a mission to craft unyielding bones that will endure the trials of time.

Mind-Body Benefits of Strength Training for Seniors

Exploring the mental health and cognitive benefits of engaging in regular strength training

---

Let's dive into something that's often overlooked but holds the power to transform our golden years – strength training for seniors. As we journey through time, it becomes ever more important to maintain harmony between our mental and physical well-being. One excellent approach to accomplish this is by adopting the practice of strength training, even in our golden years. In this section, we'll explore what exactly strength training for seniors is, and more importantly, how to do it safely.

Strength Training with Safety

Safety should always be the top priority, especially for seniors diving into strength training. After all, we're aiming for improved well-being, not unnecessary risks. Now, onto the topic of safety – a crucial element when it comes to a successful strength training regimen, especially for older folks.

1. Consult Your Physician: First and foremost, you should consult with your healthcare provider before diving into any fresh fitness regimen. Doctors have the scoop on your particular health requirements and constraints, making sure you're not pushing your body too hard. They can check out your health situation and propose exercises that suit your personal necessities.

2. Qualified Trainers: These professionals understand the unique needs and limitations of older adults and can tailor a program to suit your abilities. Opt for a trainer who's well-versed in senior fitness – they understand the nuances and can tailor exercises that cater to your unique abilities. With their help, you can build a routine that's challenging yet safe.

3. Start Slow and Low: Remember, it's not a race. Start with low resistance and gradually increase the intensity as your strength and confidence grow. This approach minimizes the risk of injuries and strains. Choose resistance levels that feel manageable at first, and as you become more comfortable, gradually increase the intensity.

4. Proper Form: Your body needs to move in a coordinated and precise manner to avoid injuries. Focus on maintaining proper form during exercises. Improving your workout routine doesn't just make it more productive, it also keeps you safer. If you're uncertain about a particular exercise, feel free to consult your trainer or browse some online tutorials. It's completely okay to double-check and ensure you're nailing it!

5. Listen to Your Body: Emphasizing how crucial safety is in seniors' strength training cannot be stressed enough. Prior to delving into these exercises, or any weight training regimen as such, it's essential to pick a weight that suits your capabilities. Opt for a weight that challenges your muscles appropriately while executing the exercises. Additionally, never hesitate to seek assistance if needed!

By consulting your physician, working with a knowledgeable trainer, starting slow, maintaining proper form, and tuning in to your body's signals, you're creating a safe and effective fitness journey. It's all about enjoying the process, staying healthy, and embracing a more active lifestyle as you gracefully age.

Mind-Body Benefits

As you dive into your strength training routine, you'll start noticing some incredible mind-body benefits:

Number 1. Elevating Vitality

The journey to becoming a stronger and more vibrant version of yourself begins with strength training. As we age, our muscles tend to weaken and shrink – But regular strength training can reverse this direction. You'll feel your muscles firm up, making everyday activities a breeze. Whether it's lifting groceries or enjoying a leisurely stroll, your newfound strength will make you feel unstoppable.

Number 2. Guardians of Bone and Muscle Health

As we age, maintaining the health of our bones becomes quite crucial. Strength training is an excellent strategy to maintain the strength and density of our bones, which reduces the risk of fractures and osteoporosis. In order to maintain our balance and prevent unplanned falls, muscles are essential. Strength training not only preserves muscle mass but can also improve it, giving you the power to stand tall and walk with confidence.

Number 3. Igniting the Calorie Conundrum

Strength training revs up your metabolism like nothing else! As we age, our metabolism tends to slow down, making weight management a tad trickier. But no need to worry now because strength training boosts your resting metabolic rate. This means you'll burn calories even when you're relaxing on the couch.

Number 4. A Healthier Abdomen

The relentless battle against abdominal fat is one that many of us are familiar with, regardless of age. In old age, tackling this hurdle becomes even more important because of the natural body changes that come along with getting older. The latest studies are telling us if seniors make regular strength training a part of their routine, they could actually lose some of that stubborn belly fat. So, not only does this help seniors keep off extra pounds, but also boosts their metabolism.

Number 5. More Youthful Appearance

Engaging in a well-structured strength training routine can help in sculpting a more youthful appearance. By targeting various muscle groups, seniors can improve their muscle definition and overall body composition. Increased muscle mass not only gives a toned appearance but also helps combat the age-related loss of muscle (sarcopenia) that can lead to a decrease in functional independence.

Number 6. A Shield Against Injury:

Seniors frequently worry a lot about getting injured, which is very understandable. Because our muscles aren't as strong and our bones aren't as dense as they once were, the likelihood of suffering an injury increases as we age. When elders engage in strength training, their bones, ligaments, and tendons are protected in addition to their muscles. Older adults can significantly strengthen their body's defenses by progressively increasing greater resistance to their activities, making it much less likely that they would break a bone or suffer an injury if they fall. By enhancing balance, stability, and coordination, strength training empowers seniors to move confidently and enjoy life to the fullest.

Number 7. Empowering Immune Function

When it comes to safeguarding our health, our immune system plays a pivotal role. As we grow older, however, its efficiency tends to weaken. Participating in regular workouts that prioritize building strength has actually been proven to provide a nice little boost to the immune system. From what studies have found, keeping up with your strength training on a consistent basis can actually ramp up the production of those handy immune cells. So, if you incorporate these exercises right into your usual routine, you're pretty much arming your immune system with just what it needs.

Number 8. Elevating Emotional Well-being

The link between keeping our bodies fit and our minds sharp becomes all the more important as we step into our later years. Engaging in strength training tailored for seniors brings about some significant advantages in this aspect too. This positive shift is attributed to the release of endorphins – those awesome chemicals that contribute to feelings of happiness and reduced stress. Plus, the sense of accomplishment that comes from conquering a challenging workout can significantly bolster your self-esteem and overall mental state.

Number 9. Fostering Independence

Embracing the golden years with zest requires a foundation of independence. By regularly engaging in strength-building exercises, seniors can preserve their muscle mass, bone density, and overall physical function. This preservation plays a pivotal role in enabling them to perform daily activities with ease, from carrying groceries to ascending stairs. This newfound vigor not only keeps them active but also bolsters their self-confidence, affirming that age is no barrier to self-sufficiency.

Number 10. Balance and Stability

Navigating life's journey necessitates a strong sense of balance and stability. Engaging in exercises that target core muscles, leg muscles, and proprioceptive training significantly enhances balance. With each well-executed deadlift, squat, or plank, seniors are enhancing their ability to move confidently and with grace, mitigating the risk of falls and injuries.

Number 11. Joint Health

For seniors, joint health often becomes a pressing concern as the years roll on. Thankfully, strength training holds the baton to orchestrate joint vitality. Contrary to misconceptions, appropriate strength training can be remarkably gentle on joints, promoting the production of synovial fluid that nourishes and lubricates these pivotal connectors. By engaging in low-impact resistance exercises, seniors can bestow their joints with the gift of longevity, savoring the joys of pain-free movement.

Number 12. Reducing Stress and Anxiety

Even as we become older, life may be a bit of a thrill. Maintaining strength involves more than just working out; it also involves improving your mindset and disposition. Engaging in regular strength exercises helps your body release endorphins – those natural mood lifters that make you feel like you're dancing on cloud nine. The best part is, that these endorphins not only tackle stress but also kick anxiety to the curb.

Number 13. Boosting Brain Health

It's like giving your brain a little flex too. When you get into those resistance workouts, you're not just beefing up your biceps, but you're also giving your smarts a boost. Think of it as a mental workout – each rep you do is like a puzzle piece that fits into the bigger picture of a healthier brain. Improved memory, enhanced focus, and better decision-making.

Number 14. A Positive Relationship with Your Body

The mirror – a friend to some, a foe to many. Engaging in strength training truly forges an unshakable connection with your own body. It's not all about striving for that flawless physique; rather, it's about reveling in the remarkable capabilities of your body. Every time you hoist, every single curl, you're conveying a profound message to your very self. Strength training teaches you to appreciate the journey, embrace your progress, and fall in love with the unique vessel that carries you through life.

Number 15. Building Bonds

One of the most beautiful aspects of strength training is the sense of community it can foster. Joining a senior strength training class can introduce you to like-minded individuals who share your goals. The camaraderie and support can turn your workout sessions into enjoyable social events. A group of seniors working together, cheering each other on, and sharing those small victories.

Number 16. Enhancing Postcoronary Performance

It can enhance your cardiovascular performance, making sure your heart is pumping strong and steady. That means you can embrace postcoronary life with a spring in your step.

Number 17. Resisting Diabetes

It's a fight many of us are familiar with. By increasing insulin sensitivity, those weightlifting sessions can help you resist the clutches of diabetes. It's like giving your body armor to stand strong against this health challenge.

Number 18. Combating Cancer

Cancer IS a term that really sends shivers down our spines. While there's no foolproof way to prevent it, there are steps we can take to empower our body's defense mechanisms. Strength training, for instance, has been linked to a boosted immune system.

Number 19. Boosting Mental Well-being

Engaging in regular strength training can also work wonders for your mental well-being. Every time you conquer a new weight or set a personal best; you're releasing a surge of those feel-good endorphins.

Conclusion

There you have it – the mind-body benefits of strength training for seniors that go way beyond just physical gains. We've dug into all the good stuff that strength training brings to the table for seniors and how it can really make a difference in your day-to-day life. It's an invitation to a vibrant, active, and fulfilling life as you age gracefully. As we conclude our little chat about the incredible mind-body benefits of strength training for seniors, let's make a pact. Let's promise ourselves that we'll prioritize our well-being, nurture our bodies, and bask in the wonderful sense of accomplishment that comes with every rep and lift. After all, life is a beautiful adventure, and we want to embark on it with strength, grace, and a whole lot of spirit.

Nutrition & Hydration for Muscle Health

In our never-ending pursuit of physical health and peak performance, we typically place a high value on various activities such as strength training, cardiovascular exercises, and flexibility routines. We typically overlook diet and hydration components for the health of our muscles. This piece will look at the crucial function nutrition plays in maintaining the condition of our muscles as well as the complex connection between dehydration and effectiveness.

Dehydration Affects

Dehydration causes a reduction in blood volume, and this in turn affects how much oxygen and nutrients are delivered to your muscles. Insufficient amounts of essential nutrients may cause muscular fatigue and a decline in stamina during exercises or physical activities. The right body temperature is essential for proper muscle function. Dehydration affects your body's capacity to control temperature, increasing your risk of overheating when exercising. Muscle cramps and even heat-related disorders may result from this.

The body naturally cools itself during physical exercise by sweating. As a result, important electrolytes such as potassium, sodium, and magnesium are lost. This loss is exacerbated by dehydration, which increases susceptibility, discomfort, and cramping. Consuming enough water is critical for post-workout recovery. Dehydration can impede muscle tissue growth and repair, prolonging discomfort, and slowing muscular development.

The Importance of Nutrition for Muscle Health

While balance exercises are vital for enhancing physical stability, nutrition plays an equally important role in maintaining and building muscle health, especially for seniors.

Protein for Muscle Maintenance: Muscles are constructed of protein. Our bodies may use protein less effectively as we become older. Consequently, it's crucial to make sure that you get enough lean protein from sources like poultry, fish, beans, and tofu. This aids in maintaining strength and muscular mass.

Hydration for Muscle Function: It's important to drink enough water to maintain optimum hydration. muscular cramps and poor muscular performance might result from dehydration. To promote the health of their muscles, elders should attempt to drink adequate water each day.

Balanced Diet: By having a balanced diet, the body is certain to receive all the nutrients necessary for good health. This comprises a range of vitamins and minerals to assist muscular function, carbs for energy, and fats for general health.

Antioxidants for Recovery: Fruits and vegetables include antioxidants that assist in lowering oxidative stress, which can harm muscles. Including a variety of vibrant fruits and veggies in your diet can help with health in general and muscle rehabilitation.

What Does It Mean to Have Good Muscle Health?

Having good muscle health goes beyond just having well-defined muscles. It encompasses a variety of factors that contribute to the optimal functioning of your muscles. Here are some key aspects of good muscle health:

Powerful and long-lasting muscles are a sign of good health. This implies that you may go about your everyday activities with comfort. Flexibility and a sufficient range of motion are provided by muscles that are in good condition. Strong muscles help us stay balanced and stable, lowering our chance of falling and being hurt, especially as we age.

Your metabolism is significantly influenced by your muscles. Together with bones, muscles maintain the skeletal system. Physical activity on a regular schedule lowers the risk of osteoporosis by keeping bones healthy and dense. Correct posture supports muscular health, which reduces the probability of musculoskeletal disorders including back discomfort and misalignment.

Nutrition and Hydration for Muscle Health

Water

Water is typically overlooked when discussing muscle nourishment, yet it is the unsung star of the game. Staying hydrated is essential for general health and plays an important role in muscular function. Dehydration can cause muscular cramps and impair workout performance.

Drink around 8-10 glasses of water each day, and up your consumption on workout days to restore lost fluids. Proper hydration keeps your muscles lubricated, which helps you avoid injuries and recover more quickly.

Calcium

Calcium is not just necessary for healthy bones; it additionally serves an important function in contractions of muscles. Calcium ions are produced when your muscles get instructions to contract, enabling them to contract and create force. Incorporate calcium-rich foods like dairy products and fortified plant-based alternatives into your diet. Make sure you satisfy your daily calcium needs.

Protein

Protein is the most well-known nutrient for muscle health. It contains the amino acids required for muscle repair and development. Your muscles will not be able to recuperate and strengthen after exercise if you do not consume enough protein.

Incorporate lean protein sources and plant-based choices into your diet. The quantity of protein you require depends on your level of physical activity and goals, but a rough rule of thumb is to consume 0.8 to 1.2 grams of protein per kilogram of body weight every day.

Magnesium

While calcium facilitates muscle contraction, magnesium does the opposite – it helps muscles relax. This mineral is essential for muscular cramp prevention and general muscle function. Include magnesium-rich foods in your diet. Consider magnesium supplements if you are having difficulty fulfilling your daily requirements through diet alone, but speak with a healthcare expert first.

Vitamin D

Vitamin D is produced by your skin in reaction to being exposed to sunlight. It may be derived from some meals and supplementation. Vitamin D is necessary for muscle health because it assists in calcium absorption, which is necessary for muscular contraction and general muscle function.

Vitamin D-rich foods include fatty fish like salmon egg yolks, and fortified dairy products. Spending time outside in the sun can also help your body naturally manufacture this important component. Ensuring you have an adequate intake of Vitamin D can contribute to stronger and healthier muscles.

Glutamine

Glutamine is an amino acid that helps in muscle repair and development. It is especially good for people who engage in strenuous physical activity like weightlifting and bodybuilding. This amino acid aids in muscle restoration after severe exercises by preventing muscular breakdown.

Glutamine-rich foods include meat, fish, dairy products, and certain plant-based sources. Including these nutrients in your diet will help with muscle rehabilitation and help you reach your muscle-building objectives.

Carbohydrates

Carbohydrates are sometimes misinterpreted, although they are an essential part of any muscle-building nutrition. They offer energy for your exercises and aid in the replenishment of glycogen reserves in your muscles, ensuring they have adequate fuel for activity and recuperation.

Complex carbs, such as whole grains, oatmeal, and sweet potatoes, are good sources of long-lasting energy. To promote muscle growth and repair, you must find an appropriate balance between protein and carbs.

Potassium

Potassium is an electrolyte that is necessary for muscular function and cramp prevention. It promotes muscle contractions and aids in fluid management in the body. Maintaining proper potassium levels can increase exercise efficacy and minimize the occurrence of muscle-related disorders.

Bananas as well as other foods such as potatoes, lettuce, and legumes are also high in this vitamin. By boosting muscle health, including potassium-rich foods in your diet will help you reach your exercise objectives.

Beta-Alanine

Beta-alanine, a non-essential amino acid, is an early form of carnosine, a molecule present in your muscles. Carnosine reduces muscular exhaustion and allows you to push harder during exercises by buffering lactic acid buildup. Consuming a Beta-alanine-rich diet can boost your workout results and your muscular growth.

Iron:

Iron is a mineral that is required for the supply of oxygen to your muscles during workouts. Iron deficiency can cause muscular weakness and decreased endurance. Consuming iron-rich meals can aid in improving muscular function and general performance.

B12:

B12 is a very essential vitamin for muscle growth as it helps in the production of red blood cells, which are the main way of transporting oxygen to the muscles and the whole body. Muscle weakness and fatigue can result from a B12 shortage. Maintain excellent muscle function by eating foods high in B12.

Omega-3

Omega-3 fatty acids, in addition to vitamins and minerals, promote muscular health. Omega-3 fatty acids may aid in muscle protein synthesis, maintain a healthy inflammatory response, guard against oxidative damage, and regulate cell communication to aid in the maintenance of healthy aging muscles.

Frequently Asked Questions about Nutrition and Hydration for Muscle Health

While there is a wealth of information available on the internet, sorting through it all may be daunting. To make things easier, we've created a list of commonly asked questions concerning muscle nutrition and hydration.

Question 1: How important is food when it comes to muscle building?

Your nutrition is critical to attaining your muscle-building objectives. It's not just about pumping iron at the gym; what you eat may make or ruin your success. Muscles require sufficient nutrition and energy to develop and heal. As a result, a well-balanced diet is essential for any successful muscle-building routine.

Question 2: What are the best foods for building muscle mass quickly?

Building muscle efficiently requires a diet rich in specific nutrients. Protein, for example, is crucial because it contains the amino acids required for muscle repair and development. Lean meats like chicken and turkey, fish, eggs, and dairy items are all high in protein. Vegetarians and vegans should eat plant-based foods including beans, tofu, and quinoa. Furthermore, complex carbohydrates such as whole grains, fruits, and vegetables give the energy required for strenuous activities.

Healthy fats also contribute to muscular health by assisting with hormone synthesis and general body function. Avocados, almonds, seeds, and olive oil are all good sources of healthful fats. Don't overlook micronutrients! Vitamin D, calcium, magnesium, and zinc are all necessary for muscular contraction and general health.

Question 3: How does nutrition and hydration affect muscle recovery?

Proper nutrition and hydration are essential for muscle recovery. Muscles require nutrition after vigorous activity to heal and get stronger. Post-workout protein and carbohydrate consumption can assist in replacing glycogen levels and deliver the amino acids required for muscle repair. Staying hydrated promotes speedier recovery by assisting in the elimination of metabolic waste products.

Question 4: How Does an Athlete's Diet Differ from a Regular Person's Diet?

Athletes' dietary needs are distinct owing to the higher physical demands they make on their bodies. Athletes usually need extra calories to fuel their energy expenditure during training and performance. This involves consuming more calories per day than someone who has a sedentary lifestyle.

Protein is crucial for muscle repair and growth. Athletes need more protein to repair muscle damage caused by intense training sessions. Athletes' protein consumption is often higher than that of ordinary people. Carbohydrates are the body's principal energy source. Athletes frequently take more carbs to fuel their exercises and assist in recuperation. Athletes must stay hydrated since even minor dehydration might affect performance. They need to replenish fluids lost through sweat during exercise.

Question 5: How to Train with Low Carbohydrate Availability

Training with low carbohydrate availability is a strategy used by some athletes to enhance endurance and fat utilization. This approach, often referred to as "train low," involves performing workouts with reduced carbohydrate stores.

Question 6: Why Do Macronutrients Matter?

Macronutrients, or carbs, proteins, and lipids, are the building blocks of a healthy diet. They are necessary for muscular health and general wellness. Carbohydrates, as previously stated, are the major energy source. They give rapid energy for exercises and aid in the maintenance of glycogen reserves throughout extended activity.

Proteins are the structural components of muscular tissue. Consuming enough protein is essential for muscle repair and development. Protein is used by people to recuperate from tough activities. Fats provide additional energy, particularly during low-intensity, long-duration activities. They also play a function in hormone production and general wellness.

Conclusion

Incorporating exercises for balance into one's daily life and eating healthy meals are vital steps to keep and improve muscle fitness. These strategies not only improve physical stability but also assist us in living a better life as we age. It is never too late to begin concentrating on muscle health with an integrated approach to exercise and food.

Importance of Staying Hydrated

We often underestimate the power of a simple yet vital habit: staying hydrated. It might seem like a small thing, but ensuring your body gets enough water can make a huge difference in your overall health. In this article, we'll dive into the many perks of staying hydrated and why it should be a cornerstone of your wellness routine.

The Foundation for Improved Health

Hydration, in all its simplicity, serves as the foundation for a healthier you. By maintaining a balanced hydration level, you're setting the stage for numerous bodily functions to work harmoniously. From regulating body temperature to keeping your joints well-lubricated, every sip of water plays a part in preventing infections, delivering essential nutrients to your cells, and sustaining the proper functioning of your organs.

Enhanced Cognitive Function and Mood

Yet, the significance of hydration doesn't stop at the physical level. Science tells us that staying well-hydrated has a direct correlation with enhanced cognitive functions and mood upliftment. Quality sleep, a sharper mind, and a brighter mood become your allies on the journey to a more fulfilling life.

Personalized Hydration Goals

Many people still find it reasonable to follow the conventional wisdom and consume 6 to 8 glasses of water each day. Each person has different preferences! Our bodies have different needs and signals when it comes to hydration. For most individuals, listening to your body and quenching your thirst should suffice in maintaining proper hydration. Some might thrive on less than the conventional 8 glasses, while others might require more.

Hydration from Nature's Bounty

While the benefits of water are undeniable, nature offers alternative ways to stay hydrated. Fruits and vegetables like watermelon, tomatoes, and lettuce are not just culinary delights but also hidden reservoirs of hydration. Sipping on herbal teas, nutrient-rich milk, or the pure goodness of fruit and vegetable juices can also contribute to your daily hydration tally.

Steer Clear of the Sugary Trap

Be careful of your decisions as you set out on your quest for greater hydration. Although sugar-sweetened beverages may be appealing, they might hinder your progress by adding extra calories and possibly dangerous ingredients. Opting for natural, unsweetened sources of hydration is your best bet.

Link of Hydration and Caffeine

This natural stimulant, commonly present in coffee, tea, and even certain soft drinks, is renowned for delivering a quick energy surge. But let's not forget, caffeine also has a role in the hydration game. While it offers its own set of advantages, it's crucial to remember its impact on our hydration status. Caffeine, often hanging out in our morning coffee and select teas, could make us visit the restroom more frequently. This uptick in bathroom breaks might accidentally edge us towards dehydration if we're not careful. What's more, caffeine can occasionally spark feelings of jitteriness or unease – quite a contrast to the serene feeling of a well-hydrated body. Regularly enjoying moderate amounts of caffeine usually won't turn into dehydration, especially when we're teaming it up with good old water intake.

Benefits of Hydration:

I totally get that you've probably come across this advice a bunch of times already, but seriously, there's a whole world of reasons beyond just satisfying your thirst. Here are some awesome perks of staying hydrated that might just give you that extra nudge to make drinking water a daily habit!

Number 1. Boosting Brain Power

Have you ever experienced those moments when your mind gets all fuzzy, and focusing on anything becomes a struggle? Well, it's possible that your brain cells are giving you a signal – they're really craving some hydration. Giving your brain the right amount of water directly affects how well it functions. Optimal hydration enables your brain cells to communicate smoothly, resulting in sharper cognitive abilities. This means improved concentration, a more agile memory, and quicker thinking.

Number 2. A Hydrated Body is a Peak-Performing Body

Hydration doesn't just influence your brain – it affects your physical performance too. You're on the treadmill, and suddenly your muscles decide to stage a cramp-fest. Chances are, they're letting you know they're running low on the hydration they need to work seamlessly. Staying hydrated helps balance the important electrolytes that keep your muscles contracting smoothly, producing energy, and generally performing at their best. So, whether you're crushing it at the gym or simply navigating through your daily routine, that water bottle of yours should never be far.

Number 3. Nourishing the Joints:

Let's dive into something that's relevant for both the spry and the not-so-spry – joint health. Think of your joints as the hinges that keep your body moving. Just like any hinge, they work better with a little lubrication. This is where hydration steps in. The cartilage in your joints receives the nutrition it requires when you are adequately hydrated, ensuring that your joints function smoothly and painlessly. Therefore, bear in mind that every drink you take is a step towards happier, more flexible joints.

Number 4. Nurturing Your Inner Wellness

Visualizing your body as a finely tuned mechanism. Just as you wouldn't take your car on the road with an empty tank, treating your body to adequate water is equally vital. Drinking plenty of water is essential for maintaining your digestive system's optimal performance. Your digestive tract can effectively process meals and absorb all those essential nutrients when your body is adequately hydrated. It's akin to equipping your body with the right instruments to lay a solid groundwork for robust health.

Number 5. Your Natural Headache Remedy

Who hasn't experienced the pounding discomfort of a headache? Before you reach for that painkiller, consider this – dehydration could be the culprit. When you're low on water, your brain can temporarily contract or shrink from fluid loss. The result? Your brain pulling away from your skull, and hello, headache. When your hydration levels are ample, your blood becomes an efficient transporter of oxygen to your cells, furnishing you with the verve needed to conquer your day. By sipping on water throughout the day, you're giving your brain the cushion it needs to stay headache-free.

Number 6. Oxygenating Your Body

Your blood acts as a messenger, bringing all kinds of treats to every part of your body. Now, what's the most important cargo it's carrying? Oxygen! And guess what? Water is like the highway that helps this precious cargo reach its destination. When you're well-hydrated, your blood can easily transport oxygen to your cells, giving you the energy you need to conquer the day.

Number 7. Radiant Skin

Move over, expensive skincare products – there's a new beauty secret in town, and it's as simple as raising a glass. Well-hydrated skin equals happy skin, and here's the rationale: water actively preserves your skin's elasticity, leading to fewer appearance of fine lines and wrinkles. Additionally, it assists in expelling toxins, resulting in a complexion that exudes freshness and radiance. Thus, prior to splurging on that exorbitant serum, ensure you're granting your skin the hydration it yearns for.

Number 8. Hydration and the Journey of Weight Management

Did you ever stop to think that staying hydrated could also play a part here? Yes, you heard it correctly! Hydration can actually give your metabolism a little nudge. When you're properly hydrated, your body's cells perform at their best, and that includes your metabolism doing its thing just right. Plus, our brains sometimes mix up thirst with hunger, causing us to snack when all we really need is a good gulp of water. So, whether you're aiming to shed a bit of weight or maintain where you're at, keep in mind that having water by your side throughout the day can be your subtle supporter.

Number 9. Linking Hydration and Temperature Regulation

Staying hydrated can be like having your own personal temperature control. Our bodies use sweat to cool down, and guess what makes up a big part of sweat? You guessed it – water. When you're well-hydrated, your body has what it needs to produce sweat effectively and keep you cool. But if dehydration shows up, the risk of heat-related troubles like heat exhaustion and heatstroke can rise.

Number 10. Electrolytes

These tiny, electrically charged particles might not always steal the show, but they're major players in our body's story. Electrolytes are the keepers of fluid balance, both inside and outside our cells. Think of them as little guardians, ensuring that everything stays where it should. When you're keeping hydrated, your electrolyte levels usually stay in harmony, allowing your muscles, nerves, and all sorts of bodily functions to operate smoothly. Yet, when dehydration steps in, the equilibrium gets disrupted, opening the door to cramps, fatigue, and a range of not-so-pleasant experiences.

Number 11. Boosting Heart Health

It's not simply a matter of drinking water; it's about providing your heart with the hydration it craves to work at its best. When you keep yourself well-hydrated, your blood flows more smoothly, helping your heart circulate it throughout your entire body with less effort. This might even lower the chances of facing heart-related problems in the future. Your heart will surely thank you for the extra care!

Number 12. Guarding Against Kidney Stone

Did you know that staying hydrated is like having a secret weapon against these pesky stones? When you keep your fluid intake up, you're helping to dilute the concentration of minerals and salts in your urine. This makes it less likely for those notorious kidney stones to form. It's like nature's way of saying, "Here's a simple solution to a not-so-simple problem!" So, raise your water bottles and toast to your kidney health – those stones won't know what hit 'em!

Number 13. Your Natural Hangover Shield

We've all been there – a night of celebration that leads to a morning of regret. Hangovers are not fun, but the good news is that you can take steps to prevent or at least minimize their wrath. Yep, you guessed it – by staying hydrated! Alcohol is known to cause your body to become dehydrated, which is one of the main causes of the throbbing headaches and nausea you experience after a night of drinking. But if you drink water wisely, you can give your body a chance. You're aiding your body in eliminating toxins and preventing hangover symptoms by sipping water in between those pricey cocktails. It's like having a magical shield that wards off the morning-after blues!

Number 14. Enhanced Detoxification

Do you know that feeling of satisfaction when you gulp down a glass of water after a workout or a long day? Well, that's your body thanking you for giving it the means to detoxify. Staying hydrated helps your kidneys do their job – flushing out waste and toxins from your system. Think of it as a mini spa day for your inner organs, helping them function at their best and ensuring that waste doesn't hang around longer than it should.

Number 15. How Hydration Aids Waste Removal

If your body were a well-oiled machine, water would be the lubricant that keeps everything operating efficiently. Maintaining a healthy level of hydration maintains your body's natural equilibrium and keeps bodily processes like digestion and circulation running smoothly. It's like pressing the system's reset button, enabling waste products from metabolism and cellular processes to be effectively flushed out. A body that is properly hydrated is like a blank slate that is prepared to handle everything life throws at it.

Number 16. Hydration and Exercise

If you're someone who loves to break a sweat at the gym or enjoys a good jog in the park, listen up – staying hydrated can seriously level up your exercise game. Dehydration can lead to decreased endurance, reduced coordination, and a dip in overall performance. When you're properly hydrated, your body can regulate its temperature more effectively, ensuring you don't overheat during that intense spin class or weightlifting session.

Conclusion

In a world bustling with complex health regimes and fitness trends, the simplicity of hydration often goes unnoticed. But remember, it's the small, consistent efforts that lay the groundwork for significant change. By prioritizing hydration, you are paving the way for improved physical health, heightened cognitive function, and a sunnier disposition. So, raise your glass – to health, vitality, and the remarkable benefits of staying hydrated.

Easing Joint Pain Through Strength Training

Exploring How Properly Designed Strength Training Routines Can Alleviate Joint Discomfort

---

Let's discuss joint discomfort, a subject that many of us can relate to, and how we may combat it by utilizing the incredible realm of strength training. We are all aware of how challenging managing joint pain can be, particularly if you have arthritis. But what if I told you that, while initially seeming paradoxical, weightlifting may really be a game-changer in managing arthritis and improving your general quality of life?

Strength Training with Joint Pain: Is It Good or Bad for You?

Weightlifting with arthritis sounds like a disaster, right? You see, the response isn't as straightforward as just saying "yes" or "no." It actually relies on your strategy for handling the situation. Without the proper instruction, starting to carry big objects might make your joint discomfort worse. However, and this is the intriguing part, weightlifting can really aid in the battle against arthritis if you are wise about it and adopt a balanced approach.

Lifting weights may be quite beneficial for your joints if you do it correctly and have an expert coach you through it. How? Consider it this way: moving your joints through their whole range of motion, even with just a little weight, helps to lubricate them and reduce stiffness.

Your muscles grow stronger as you lift weights. And that strength? It's like a support system for your joints. Imagine having a backup crew that takes some of the pressure off your joints during your regular activities. That, my friend, could mean less pain and more ability to move around. It's like giving your joints a friendly hand to help them do their job better.

How to avoid joint pain during strength training?

It's simple to get carried away and go all out when it comes to strength training. Your body, however, is the best teacher here. Keep an eye out for the cues it gives you. It's fine to back off a little if a certain movement doesn't seem quite right or if you feel any pain. Keep in mind that everybody is different, so what suits one person may not be the greatest for you.

Tip 1: The Essential Warm-Up

This crucial step often gets skipped in the rush to get to the heavy lifting. Believe me, your joints will thank you for not bypassing this important prelude. A good warm-up does more than simply raise your heart rate. It genuinely helps to limber up your joints, getting them all set for the weightlifting session ahead. Take around 5-10 minutes for some dynamic stretches and easy cardio to get your blood circulating and your joints ready to roll.

Tip 2: The Post-Lifting Stretch

Always make sure to engage in some post-lifting stretches. Stretching out those worked muscles helps ease any tension that might be causing joint discomfort. The key is to focus on both the muscles and the joints that were heavily involved in your session. Hold each stretch for around 15-30 seconds and breathe through it – your joints will sigh in relief.

Tip 3: A Slow and Steady Approach to Adding Weight

Gradually increasing the weight you lift gives your joints and connective tissues the chance to adapt without feeling like they're taking on too much too soon. Think of it as a marathon, not a sprint – your joints will stay happier for it.

Tip 4: Embrace the Mix-Up in Your Routine

If joint pain is giving you grief, consider introducing some variety into your workout routine. Alternate between different exercises that work the same muscle groups – this can help distribute the stress across various joints, preventing overuse and reducing the likelihood of discomfort. Plus, mixing things up keeps your workouts fresh and exciting!

Tip 5: The Art of Form Focus

As you venture into the world of strength training, never underestimate the power of proper form. Trust me, your joints are the first ones to notice if your form is off. Whether it's a deadlift, a squat, or a bench press, prioritize maintaining correct alignment and posture. This not only optimizes muscle engagement but also ensures that your joints are moving in a way that's biomechanically sound, minimizing unnecessary strain.

Benefits of Strength Training for Easing Joint Pain

1: Flexibility and Freedom

When your joints just don't want to cooperate and every movement seems like a chore. Well, weightlifting could be your friend to loosen up those surly joints. As you engage in regular strength training, your muscles start to become stronger, helping to stabilize and support your joints. This added muscular support can ease the strain on your joints, reducing pain and stiffness. Plus, the dynamic movements involved in weight lifting promote flexibility, making it easier for you to move around without wincing at every step.

2: Boosts Bone Health

As we grow older, our bones might become a tad more fragile, which isn't the best update for those of us coping with arthritis. Nevertheless, worry not, as weightlifting can step in to help once more! When you partake in weight-bearing activities, such as lifting weights, you're essentially giving your bones a purpose to toughen up. This is of particular significance for folks with arthritis, as sturdy bones offer enhanced backing to the impacted joints. So, on your next visit to the gym, keep in mind that you're not solely lifting weights – you're also elevating your bone well-being!

3: Weight Lifting and Weight Management

One of the key factors in managing joint pain is maintaining a healthy weight. Lugging around those extra pounds might just add some strain to your joints, making things even more uncomfortable. But no worries, diving into weightlifting could truly shake things up on your quest to handle your weight. When you regularly dive into strength training, you're not just constructing muscle, you're cranking up your metabolism too. What that boils down to is your body becoming a whiz at torching calories, ultimately giving you a hand in ditching those unwanted pounds. Less weight equals less stress on your joints, leading to fewer aches and an overall improved quality of life.

4. Strengthening the Muscles that Guard Your Joints:

When you engage in weight lifting, you're essentially working these muscles, making them stronger and more resilient. This enhanced muscular support directly contributes to reducing joint pain. When your muscles are in top form, they help share the load that your joints bear. This redistribution of stress takes some of the pressure off your joints, making movement smoother and less painful.

5. Fostering Better Balance:

Weight lifting helps train your muscles to work in harmony, which in turn improves your overall balance. As your balance gets better, you're less likely to experience falls or awkward movements that could worsen your joint pain.

6. Boosting Blood Flow and Nutrient Delivery:

When you engage in strength training, your body responds by increasing blood flow to the worked muscles. This surge in blood flow brings along a host of goodies, including essential nutrients and oxygen. Now, why is this important for easing joint pain? Enhanced blood circulation leads to a heightened nutrient supply to your joints, supporting their repair and recovery processes effectively. This can play a significant role in diminishing inflammation and fostering the healing process, both of which play a pivotal role in effectively managing the discomfort caused by arthritis. In essence, engaging in strength training prepares the perfect platform for your body's innate healing mechanisms to take action, providing much-needed support to your joints.

The Importance of a Discussing with Your Doctor First:

A heart-to-heart discussion with your healthcare practitioner is essential. Why? We all have different medical histories, physical ailments, and underlying health problems. What is perfect for one individual may not be appropriate for another. Your fitness journey will be customized to your unique needs if you share your objectives with your doctor. They can provide insights into the types of exercises that would be safe and beneficial for your joints.

Unlocking the Power of Strengthening Exercises:

These workouts are made to target particular muscle groups that surround your joints and provide that support. Building muscular strength effectively relieves some of the pressure on your joints, allowing for easier and more comfortable movement.

Walking Your Way to Comfort

Let's begin our joint-saving journey with something as simple as putting one foot in front of the other – walking! Walking is an excellent low-impact exercise that gets your blood flowing and your joints moving without subjecting them to undue stress. A brisk walk around your neighborhood or a leisurely stroll in the park can do wonders for your joint mobility.

Aerobic Exercise

While we're on the subject of joint-friendly exercises, let's not forget about the wonders of aerobic workouts. They aren't just about getting your heart pumping; they can also be gentle on your joints. Think about low-impact options like swimming, stationary cycling, or brisk walking. These activities get your blood flowing and your joints moving without subjecting them to unnecessary strain.

Range-of-Motion Exercises

Think of them as your daily dose of stretching and flexibility training. Yoga and tai chi are fantastic examples – they're a delicate balance of strength, flexibility, and mindfulness. Your joints will thank you for these graceful movements that encourage fluidity and help prevent stiffness.

Stretching

The age-old remedy for tight muscles and aching joints. Incorporating gentle stretches into your routine can work wonders in alleviating joint pain. Think about it as giving your joints a little TLC. Stretching helps improve flexibility and range of motion, both of which are crucial for joint health. Spend a few minutes each day performing simple stretches, focusing on the areas that give you trouble.

Serenity of Swimming

Immersing yourself in the soothing embrace of water, where your joints can experience true weightlessness. Swimming is a fantastic exercise for joint pain relief, as the buoyancy of the water eliminates impact and allows you to move without stressing your joints. Whether it's doing laps, water aerobics, or simply enjoying a leisurely swim, you'll be amazed at how your joints thank you for this aquatic escape.

Weight Bearing Exercises

Weight-bearing exercises can be your secret weapon against joint pain. These workouts require you to use your muscles against gravity, which allows your joints to adapt and strengthen. The weight-bearing activities squats, lunges, and even push-ups are excellent examples. You can help your body build the strength it needs to support your joints by performing these exercises.

Cycling

It is an underrated exercise. Not only does it give your heart a good workout, but it's also gentle on your joints. The way cycling's fluid motion glides along actually boosts the circulation to your joints. That, in turn, might help ease up that stiffness and bothersome ache.

Conclusion

So, there you go, everyone. Although it's undoubtedly an excellent thing bulking up and having an enviable physique aren't the only benefits of weight lifting. It's about giving yourself the authority to take charge of the health of your joints, especially if you have arthritis. You may help your body fight the effects of arthritis by increasing bone strength through weight-bearing workouts, reducing joint pain and stiffness, and increasing joint mobility.

Of course, as with any exercise program, it's imperative to speak with your doctor before starting a weightlifting program, especially if you have any pre-existing ailments. Weight lifting, however, can be a fun path toward a healthier, more active, and more comfortable existence with the appropriate direction and strategy. So, let's lift those weights and ease that joint pain together!

Choosing the Right Exercises

Low-impact and Joint-Friendly Exercises Suitable for Seniors

In our fast-paced modern world, taking care of our health is a big deal. And one key ingredient in the recipe for feeling great is staying active through regular workouts. But with so many exercise options out there, how do we choose what's right for us? Well, in this piece, we're going to explore the perks of workouts that are gentle on our joints, how staying active can help us stay healthy, and how regular exercise gives our brain a real boost.

Low-Impact Workouts: A Gentle Approach to Fitness

The best thing about these routines is that they keep you fit without going hard on your joints. Basically, these workouts involve moves that are easy on your bones and joints. No matter your level of fitness, age, or whether you're recovering from an ailment, this makes them a win for everyone. If you're thinking of low-impact workouts, you can consider walking, cycling, yoga, and swimming.

What's really great is that these workouts are chill enough that you won't push yourself too far. So, if you're all about staying active but not looking for a trip to Overexertion City, this is your jam. Especially if you're starting out on your fitness journey, these exercises are gold. They're all about the long game – keeping you moving without the whole injury risk thing.

Exercise as a Shield Against Disease

Apart from the immediate perks of boosting your energy and keeping a balanced weight, incorporating regular exercise can have a profound impact on your overall well-being and lifespan. The realm of scientific studies highlights how exercise takes on a pivotal role in safeguarding you against an array of illnesses. Whether it's heart conditions, type 2 diabetes, or even specific forms of cancer, physical activity steps up as a defender, aiding your body in repelling these potential health hazards.

The magic of exercise extends to your cardiovascular system by refining circulation, fortifying your heart muscles, and steadying blood pressure levels. What's more, it elevates your immune system's prowess to combat infections while curbing inflammation - a shared root cause in numerous chronic ailments.

Boosting Brain Function Through Physical Activity

Even though we are all aware of the benefits exercise has for our bodies, it's amazing how much it also benefits our minds. It has been demonstrated that including regular physical activity in your routine might enhance brain function. It's like a workout for your mind!

So, when you get moving, your body lets out these tiny chemicals called neurotransmitters. These guys, like dopamine and serotonin, are famous for being the mood regulators that also help us chill out. And guess what? They don't just keep our spirits high; they also help our brain handle info like a champ. Cool, right?

Experts even found out that exercise can spark the birth of new brain cells. It's like a party for your brain, encouraging it to be flexible and sharp. And who doesn't want a sharp brain? So, the next time you're breaking a sweat, just remember, you're doing a solid for your brain too.

17 Low-Impact Exercises for Seniors

1. Walking

Strolling on foot is truly an underestimated form of exercise. It's a classic undertaking that is kind to your joints and highly beneficial for your heart's well-being. Engaging in regular walks doesn't merely contribute to your cardiac health; it also presents an opportunity to immerse yourself in nature, declutter your thoughts, and even engage socially with companions. Whether you're taking a relaxed saunter around the local area or embarking on a spirited walk in the park, the simple act of putting one foot in front of the other can perform miracles for your comprehensive physical condition. Furthermore, it conveniently provides a valid reason to bask in some nourishing Vitamin D courtesy of the sun!

2. Chair Yoga

Sit into a comfortable chair as you flow through a series of gentle poses and stretches. Chair yoga is like a soothing journey for your body. It's all about boosting your flexibility, balance, and posture while respecting what your body can do. Especially great for older folks who might find regular yoga a bit challenging or for anyone wanting a laid-back way to stay fit. So, why not get yourself a chair and start this wonderful adventure towards finding your inner calm and feeling refreshed?

3. Barre

You won't need a dance background to excel at this exercise. Barre workouts typically involve a combination of ballet-inspired movements, light weights, and a sturdy support to hold onto (no tutus required!). These exercises focus on enhancing muscular strength, flexibility, and stability. Plus, they're a fantastic way to engage your core muscles and maintain a strong posture.

4. Aqua Adventures

When it comes to a low-impact and joint-friendly exercise, water aerobics emerges as a true winner. The way the water supports you really eases up on your joints, all while giving you some pushback for a solid all-around session. This makes it a really nice option for folks dealing with things like arthritis or achy joints. And it's not just about the body – doing aerobics in the water lets you connect with others too, since group classes often build up a sense of togetherness. The water's calming vibe, mixed with the sense of camaraderie, can turn a workout into a bit of a revitalizing escape rather than just another task.

5. Resistance Band Routines

Building and maintaining muscle strength is of paramount importance, especially as we age. Resistance band workouts offer an incredibly versatile way to achieve this. These elastic bands provide gentle resistance, helping to enhance muscle strength without putting unnecessary stress on the joints. From seated leg lifts to seated rows, there's a wide range of exercises that can be tailored to individual needs. Furthermore, resistance bands are lightweight and portable, making them a convenient option for staying active at home or while traveling.

6. Pilates

Pilates, often referred to as "the art of controlled movements," is a great exercise option for seniors aiming to improve their core strength and flexibility. Pilates focuses on controlled breathing, smooth and precise movements, and mindful concentration. This not only helps in building a strong core but also aids in maintaining better posture. The gentle and deliberate nature of Pilates makes it suitable for seniors with varying fitness levels, allowing each individual to progress at their own pace.

7. Yoga

Amidst the chaos of modern life, Yoga stands as a beacon of tranquility and wellness. This age-old technique not only takes care of your physical needs but also develops your intellect. Yoga aims to strike a balance between your physical and mental well-being via a sequence of postures, regulated breathing, and meditation. Yoga's versatility is what makes it so beautiful. Whether you're a seasoned practitioner or a complete novice, there's a Yoga style that suits your needs. From the dynamic flow of Vinyasa to the precise alignment of Iyengar, each style offers a unique experience. Yoga enhances flexibility, builds muscular endurance, and even aids in stress reduction.

8. Tai Chi

Originating in ancient China, Tai Chi is often referred to as a "moving meditation." The graceful, fluid movements of Tai Chi not only promote physical fitness but also foster mental clarity. Often practiced in serene outdoor settings, Tai Chi combines slow, deliberate movements with deep breathing, creating a harmonious synergy. Tai chi's primary goals are internal harmony and balance. It strengthens muscles, increases flexibility, and improves posture. It is a low-impact workout. Tai Chi is a great option for people looking for a comprehensive approach to exercise because of its relaxing and stress-relieving soft, flowing movements.

9. Seated Hamstring Stretch

This gentle yet effective stretch is like a warm hug for your leg muscles. It's fantastic for flexibility and takes mere minutes to do. Here's how it goes: You sit comfortably, extend one leg, and lean forward slightly from your hips. It's like reaching for your toes, but with a relaxed vibe. You'll feel the gentle pull in the back of your thigh, which is your hamstring giving you a friendly nod of approval. Hold it for a few deep breaths, switch sides, and voilà! You've just embraced an exercise that feels amazing and keeps you limber.

10. Gardening

Now, let's step outside into the sun-soaked haven of your backyard. Gardening isn't just about cultivating beautiful flowers and fresh veggies; it's also a fantastic way to sneak in some exercise without even realizing it. All that digging, planting, and weeding might as well be a full-body workout. Bending down to plant those seeds? That's like a mini squat right there. Reaching for those high branches? Your arms and shoulders are getting a solid stretch. Even lugging around bags of soil can be compared to weightlifting – minus the intimidating equipment.

11. Cycling

Whether you're pedaling through your neighborhood or enjoying scenic trails, cycling is a fantastic way to get your heart pumping while exploring your surroundings. Hop on your bike and feel the wind in your hair (don't forget that helmet, though – safety first!). It's an exercise that's gentle on your joints and offers a great cardiovascular workout. Plus, you can tailor your cycling intensity to match your fitness level and goals. So, dust off that bike, hop on and relive those carefree moments while getting fit.

12. Squats with Alternate Reach

Squats with Alternate Reach, a move that adds a delightful twist to the traditional squat. As you lower yourself into a squat, reach out with one arm, as if you're aiming for the stars. By strengthening your balance and using your core, this straightforward addition gives your workout a new depth.

13. Strength Training

Strength training is the key to shaping your physique and packing on some significant muscle. This is more about increasing your general strength and energy than it is about becoming a bodybuilder (unless that is your aim, of course). It's similar to giving your body a tune-up so it can easily face problems in daily life.

14. Rowing

Rowing isn't just for competitive athletes or water enthusiasts. It's an intense, whole-body workout. Rowing is a fantastic exercise for burning calories while experiencing the impression of floating on water because its rhythmic action works your arms, legs, and core. Plus, the low-impact nature of rowing is gentle on your joints, giving you a great workout without unnecessary strain.

15. The Balance Beam

The balance beam might not be the first thing that comes to mind for a workout, but it's an excellent tool for enhancing your core strength and stability. Walking across a balance beam challenges your body to engage numerous muscles simultaneously. It's like a tightrope act that enhances your coordination and balance, all while keeping your muscles guessing.

16. Cat-Camel Stretch

Flexibility and mobility are essential aspects of fitness that often take a back seat. Enter the cat-camel stretch, a simple yet highly effective exercise to keep your spine supple and your back muscles relaxed. As you move through the arching and rounding motions, you're giving your spine a much-needed stretch, while also encouraging better posture and relieving tension.

17. The Single-Leg Stand

Balance is a cornerstone of functional fitness. The single-leg stand might seem basic, but it's a powerhouse move for enhancing your stability. By standing on one leg, you're engaging your core, activating small stabilizing muscles, and training your body to distribute weight evenly. It's a fantastic exercise for preventing injuries and improving your overall balance and coordination.

Conclusion

The appropriate workouts may make all the difference in the pursuit of a better lifestyle. Low-impact exercises are a great option for people of all fitness levels since they offer a gentle and sustainable method of remaining active. Additionally, exercise helps your body ward against dangers and preserve optimum health as a great disease prevention strategy. Regular physical activity has advantages that go beyond the physical sphere since it enhances mental health and cognitive function.

Progressive Overload and Adaptation

Welcome to a journey where muscle meets mastery, and sweat transforms into strength. Today, we're diving into the fascinating world of Progressive Overload and Adaptation, the twin pillars of fitness progress. It's not just lifting weights; it's a dynamic dance between pushing your limits and letting your body evolve. Buckle up, as we explore how this simple yet profound concept can reshape your fitness journey, one rep at a time.

What is Progressive Overload?

Progressive overload is a simple concept. It's all about gradually increasing the demand you place on your muscles over time. Our bodies are pretty smart – they adapt to challenges to become more efficient. It describes the overtime steady rise in exercise intensity, duration, or frequency. Simply said, it's about pushing your physical boundaries and discovering new methods to test your body. The concept is applicable to all forms of exercise, including yoga, swimming, jogging, and weightlifting.

You're lifting weights. If you consistently lift the same weight, your muscles will adapt and your growth will stagnate, even if you first feel comfortable doing so. Progressive overload enters the frame in this situation. Lifting heavier weight over time forces your muscles to work harder, adapt, and get stronger.

Periodization

Periodization is the strategic manipulation of training variables over distinct periods of time. Think of it as a dynamic roadmap guiding you through different phases of training. The goal is to prevent plateaus and optimize gains by deliberately varying the intensity, volume, and type of exercises within a training cycle.

Periodization typically encompasses three main phases:

1. **Foundation Phase:** This initial stage sets the stage for progression. It emphasizes creating a strong foundation of technique, stability, and strength. The volume is doable and the intensity is mild.

2. **Strength and Hypertrophy Phase:** The emphasis now is on doing moderate repetitions with stronger weights. The goal is to challenge the muscles and stimulate growth.

3. **Peaking Phase:** As you near the end of the cycle, the intensity reaches its peak. The volume decreases, allowing the body to recover while still maintaining strength and performance gains.

By cycling through these phases strategically, the body is kept in a constant state of adaptation, preventing it from becoming complacent and leading to continuous improvements.

Why Progressive Overload Matters?

If you want to truly transform your body and make strides toward your fitness goals, you've got to give it a reason to change. This is where progressive overload comes in.

The main reason people hit the gym is often to gain muscle mass. By consistently challenging your muscles with heavier weights, you create tiny micro-tears in the muscle fibers. As your body repairs these tears, the muscles grow stronger and larger. Our bodies are remarkably adaptable. If you keep doing the same exercises with the same intensity, your progress will hit a plateau. Progressive overload prevents this by constantly challenging your body and preventing it from settling into a comfort zone.

Weight-bearing exercises, a key component of progressive overload, have been linked to improved bone density. This is crucial for preventing conditions like osteoporosis, especially as we age. Intense workouts triggered by progressive overload increase your metabolism. This means you'll burn more calories even at rest, making weight management more manageable.

Benefits of Progressive Overload Training

Muscle Growth: If you're looking to bulk up, progressive overload is your ticket to gains. By continuously pushing your muscles to handle greater resistance, you trigger microscopic muscle damage, prompting your body to rebuild and reinforce those muscles. Over time, this results in noticeable growth and increased muscle mass.

Strength Development: Whether you're an athlete or a fitness enthusiast, progressive overload is your ally in building functional strength. By gradually increasing the weight you lift, you enhance your muscle fiber recruitment and overall strength capacity. This improvement in strength not only enhances performance but also reduces the risk of injury.

Plateau Busting: Hitting a plateau is frustrating, and that's where progressive overload shines. By introducing variations in intensity and workload, you challenge your body to adapt continuously. This prevents the dreaded plateau, allowing you to keep making strides toward your goals.

Mental Resilience: Embarking on a journey of progressive overload requires commitment and discipline. As you set and achieve goals, your mental resilience and determination naturally improve. These traits transcend the gym, positively impacting various aspects of your life.

Injury Prevention: Contrary to misconceptions, progressive overload, when done with proper form and technique, is a safeguard against injuries. Strengthening muscles, tendons, and ligaments enhance joint stability, reducing the risk of strains and sprains.

Methods of Progressive Overload

At its core, progressive overload is the practice of gradually increasing the demands you place on your muscles and body during exercise sessions. This deliberate and systematic approach propels your body to adapt and grow stronger over time. There are several methods that can be employed to implement progressive overload effectively:

1. **Increase Endurance:** Endurance is the foundation of any successful training journey. To progressively overload endurance, one can extend workout durations, increase the number of repetitions, or even reduce rest periods between sets. For instance, if you're accustomed to running a certain distance, try adding an extra lap or two. This slight intensification nudges your body to adapt and build greater endurance capabilities.

2. **Increasing Resistance:** Resistance training is the gold standard for building muscle and strength. Progressive overload in this realm involves gradually increasing the weight you lift or the resistance you encounter. If you've been lifting 50 pounds during your squats, consider bumping it up to 55 or 60 pounds. This incremental approach challenges your muscles and forces them to grow stronger to accommodate the newfound stress.

3. **Increase Tempo:** The tempo at which you perform exercises plays a pivotal role in your training outcomes. Altering the tempo involves manipulating the speed at which you complete each phase of an exercise. For instance, when performing a bench press, you might slow down the eccentric (lowering) phase of the movement and then explode during the concentric (lifting) phase. This novel rhythm confuses the muscles and contributes to progressive overload.

4. **Volume Augmentation:** Your muscles are more severely challenged and encouraged to grow when the overall volume of work performed during a workout is increased by increasing the number of sets, repetitions, or both. Volume, which is made up of sets and repetitions, is a crucial factor in determining training performance. Increasing volume involves adding more sets, repetitions, or both to your workouts. If you've been doing 3 sets of 10 reps for a particular exercise, consider progressing to 4 sets of 12 reps. This method injects a fresh stimulus, propelling your body to adapt by growing more resilient.

5. **Intensity Manipulation:** This method revolves around altering the amount of weight you lift during your workouts. You could help your muscles adapt to the additional stresses imposed on them by gradually increasing the load. Increase the weight of the barbell, dumbbell, or exercise equipment you're using to do a certain activity to achieve this.

6. **Increase Reps:** When it comes to progressive overload, the "more is more" philosophy may completely transform the game. By adding more repetitions to your sets, you extend the time your muscles spend under tension. This extended tension can ignite fresh muscle growth and give your body a new stimulus to adapt to.

The Limits of Progression

There are limits to how much and how quickly you can progress, even if progressive overload is a tried-and-true strategy for success. Overstepping these limits may result in injury, exhaustion, and setbacks.

The pace of improvement may slow down as your body adjusts. It's common to hit plateaus where gains become less noticeable. This is a sign that your current approach needs tweaking, not abandoning. Pushing yourself too hard and too often can lead to insufficient recovery time, impeding progress and increasing the risk of injuries.

Each person's body responds uniquely to training. What takes one individual only a little time may take another person much longer. It's crucial to pay attention to your body's signals and modify your strategy as necessary.

The Limits of Variation

While variation in your workout routines can keep things interesting and prevent stagnation, there's a limit to how much you should vary your exercises.

Constantly changing exercises might prevent you from consistently overloading specific muscle groups, hindering focused development. Mastering a movement takes time. Frequent changes could hinder your ability to progress in terms of skill and technique. Tracking progress becomes challenging when routines change too frequently, making it difficult to gauge the effectiveness of your methods.

Implementing Progressive Overload Safely

While the benefits of progressive overload are undeniable, it's essential to proceed with caution. Jumping into heavy lifting without proper form and technique can lead to injuries. Here are a few tips to keep in mind:

1. **Start Slowly:** If you've never worked out before, start with a weight that pushes you but yet lets you keep good technique. Gradually increase the weight as you become more comfortable.

2. **Listen to Your Body:** Something is wrong when there is pain. It's time to reevaluate your approach if you feel sudden or lingering pain when working out.

3. **Rest and Recover:** Muscles need time to repair and grow. Adequate sleep and proper nutrition play a vital role in this process.

Who Should Overload?

Progressive overload isn't solely the domain of elite athletes and bodybuilders. In fact, it's a principle that can be harnessed by individuals at various fitness levels. If your goal is to build muscle, enhance strength, or even improve endurance, the concept of gradually increasing resistance or intensity applies to you. This principle is about allowing your body to adapt to increasingly demanding stimuli over time, which ultimately leads to growth and progress.

For beginners, it's essential to establish a solid foundation of proper form and technique before diving into aggressive overloading. As you build confidence and skill, gradually incorporating small increments in weight, repetitions, or intensity will stimulate your muscles and encourage development. Likewise, intermediate and advanced athletes can reap the rewards of progressive overload by pushing their limits and consistently challenging themselves to reach new heights.

Possible Pitfalls of Overloading

Injury Risk: Over Enthusiastic individuals might be tempted to rush the process and overload too quickly. This can lead to compromised form and, consequently, an increased risk of injuries. The body needs time to adapt, and patience is key.

Plateauing: Ironically, embracing progressive overload without a well-thought-out plan can lead to plateaus in progress. When your body is subjected to the same type of overload repeatedly, it can become resistant to further adaptations. Varying your routines and incorporating different exercises can help counter this.

Burnout and Overtraining: While pushing your limits is beneficial, overloading without adequate recovery can result in burnout and overtraining. Rest is as essential as the workout itself; neglecting it can have counterproductive effects.

Mental Strain: The pursuit of ever-increasing loads can sometimes lead to mental fatigue and stress, particularly if unrealistic expectations are set.

Neglecting Other Factors: Focusing solely on overload can overshadow other essential aspects of fitness, such as nutrition, sleep, and flexibility. A holistic approach is crucial for balanced growth.

Conclusion

In a nutshell, progressive overload is like giving your muscles an invitation to a transformation party. With each new challenge you throw their way, they respond by getting bigger, stronger, and more capable. So, if you're serious about sculpting that dream physique and reaching new fitness heights, make progressive overload your workout BFF.

There you have it, pals! The lowdown on progressive overload and why it's the bee's knees for your fitness journey. Do not compare yourself to anyone else since this is your own special journey. Keep being consistent and pushing the envelope as you observe your body thrive in ways you've never seen before. Until next time, keep lifting, keep growing, and keep embracing the beautiful grind!

Balancing Cardiovascular and Strength Training

You know, the debate about whether cardio or strength training is the better exercise for overall health comes up a lot. It's a bit like choosing between apples and oranges - both have their benefits, but it can be tricky to figure out the right balance. In this section, we're going to chat about the good things that both cardio and strength training bring to the table and how you can find that sweet spot between the two for your health goals.

Cardiovascular Exercise

Cardiovascular activity, or cardio for short, is any exercise that increases your heart rate and keeps it there for an extended period of time. Examples of this include dancing, brisk walking, swimming, cycling, and running. Cardio primarily attempts to improve the performance of your cardiovascular system by strengthening your heart and lungs.

1. Heart Health: Cardio workouts are champions when it comes to improving cardiovascular health. By decreasing blood pressure, boosting cholesterol levels, and increasing cardiac function, they help lessen the risk of heart disease.

2. Calorie Burn: Cardio is your buddy if weight reduction or weight maintenance is your objective. It burns calories and can help people lose excess weight.

3. Endurance: Regular cardio training can boost your stamina, enabling you to engage in activities with less fatigue and more vitality.

It's important to understand that excessive cardio might have drawbacks, just like any training program. Overdoing it might not be the best strategy for gaining lean muscle mass because it might result in overuse issues like stress fractures or tendinitis.

Strength Training

Exercises intended to develop physical strength, size, and endurance are included in strength training. This collection of exercises includes weightlifting, bodyweight exercises including push-ups and squats, and resistance band routines. Strength training primarily aims to build muscular mass and strength.

1. Muscle Development: Strength training can help you gain lean muscle mass, which will speed up your metabolism and help you develop a more sculpted and toned body.

2. Bone Health: It offers advantages beyond those related to muscle. By increasing bone density, strength exercise helps lower the risk of osteoporosis as you age.

3. Injury Prevention: You may considerably lower your risk of injuries in daily life by building up your muscles and correcting your posture.

It's possible that strength training alone won't have the same cardiovascular advantages as aerobic workouts. When it can raise your heart rate when you exercise, it often doesn't do so for as long as cardio does.

Why Both Matter

The balance between these two types of exercise is the secret to reaching holistic health. This is why:

1. Comprehensive Fitness: An all-encompassing approach to fitness is achieved by combining cardiovascular and strength training. Gaining strength, endurance, muscular growth, and improved bone health allows you to take care of every element of your health.

2. Injury Prevention: Cardio helps with flexibility and mobility, reducing the risk of injuries during strength training. On the flip side, strength training stabilizes joints, minimizing the chance of injury during cardio activities.

3. Metabolic Efficiency: Cardio and strength training complement each other by optimizing your metabolism. Cardio burns calories during the workout, while strength training builds muscle that continues to burn calories even at rest. This synergy is a recipe for maintaining a healthy weight.

Now that we've established the importance of this balance, let's address a common concern: how does cardio interfere with muscle gain?

What Are The Main Ways Cardio Interferes With Muscle Gain?

Despite the fact that cardio has many advantages, it occasionally inhibits muscular growth. The following are the main ways that might occur:

1. Caloric Deficit: Cardio burns calories, and when done excessively, it can lead to a caloric deficit. Building muscle requires a surplus of calories to fuel growth. Gaining muscle growth becomes difficult if you constantly expend more calories than you take in.

2. Overtraining: Overtraining may result from excessive cardio, especially from high-intensity exercises. Your muscles may become catabolized as a result of overtraining, deteriorating rather than growing.

3. Energy Drain: Cardio can leave you feeling drained, reducing your overall energy and enthusiasm for strength training sessions. If you're tired from a long run or an intense spin class, you may not have the energy to lift weights effectively.

4. Protein Utilization: Cardio can increase protein utilization in the body for energy. This means that the protein you consume may be used for fuel instead of muscle repair and growth.

5. Conflicting Adaptations: Cardio and strength training can lead to conflicting adaptations within muscle fibers. Cardio may promote endurance adaptations, while strength training emphasizes hypertrophy. Striking the right balance is essential to prevent interference.

Finding the Right Balance

What subsequently is the ideal ratio of aerobic to strength exercise for optimum health? The response is based on your particular objectives and the unique requirements of your body. To assist you in finding the ideal balance, consider the following rules:

1. Weight Management: For weight management and fat loss, a balanced approach is often best. Incorporate both cardio and strength training into your routine. Start off by doing three aerobic days and two strength training days per week.

2. Muscle Building: Strength training should take precedence if gaining muscle and strength is your main objective. With one or two days of moderate-intensity cardio, try to strength train at least three to four times each week.

3 Functional Fitness: Include both cardio and strength training in your regimen for general functional fitness and injury avoidance. You may increase your strength, stamina, and flexibility with the aid of this combo.

4. Pay Attention to Your Body: Above all, be aware of how your body reacts. Adjust your regimen if you're experiencing unexpected discomfort, soreness, or weariness. Any exercise routine must include rest and recuperation time.

Benefits of a Balanced Approach

Combining the two types of exercise increases your resting metabolic rate while also helping you to grow muscle and burn more calories throughout your activity. Cardio exercises improve general endurance while strengthening your heart and lungs, lowering your risk of heart disease.

Strength training sculpts your body and creates definition, while also improving your posture. A balanced routine helps you perform everyday tasks more easily and with reduced risk of injury. Exercise releases endorphins, reducing stress and improving mood.

The Difference Between Cardio and Strength Training

Cardiovascular exercise, sometimes referred to as "cardio," focuses primarily on your cardiovascular system, which includes your heart and lungs. It comprises repeated, rhythmic movements that quicken breathing and increase heart rate. While strength training focuses on employing resistance to grow and tone muscles. Lifting weights, utilizing resistance bands, or even just your body weight can do this.

Building a Strength and Cardio Routine

1. Assess Your Goals

It's critical to establish your fitness objectives prior to beginning any exercise program. Are you attempting to improve your general health, reduce your weight, put on muscle, or increase your endurance? Knowing your objectives might help you design a routine that is specific to your needs.

2. Create a Balanced Schedule

Cardiovascular and strength training should both be a part of a well-rounded fitness regimen.

- **Cardiovascular Training:** Cardio workouts are great for improving endurance and burning calories. Running, cycling, swimming, and dancing all increase heart rate and improve lung capacity. According to the American Heart Association, you should strive to do at least 150 minutes of moderate-intensity cardio or 75 minutes of vigorous-intensity cardio per week.

- **Strength training,** on the other hand, enhances general body strength while assisting in the growth of muscle. This can include resistance band exercises, bodyweight activities, or weightlifting. At least two days of strength training per week should focus on the main muscle groups.

3. Mix It Up

Variety is the flavor of life, and the same is true of your exercise program. Avoid falling into a rut by switching up your exercise routine. This may result in boredom as well as your body adapting and your development perhaps plateauing. Incorporate different types of cardio and strength exercises to keep things interesting and challenge your body in new ways.

4. Listen to Your Body

As crucial as it is to stick to your regimen, it's also critical to pay heed to your body's cues. Rest when necessary, and avoid overexerting oneself to the point of harm. For the growth of muscles and general health, adequate rest and recuperation are essential.

5. Nutrition and Hydration

Exercise alone won't yield optimal results. A balanced diet rich in nutrients and proper hydration are essential to support your fitness goals. To be sure you're providing your body with enough food for your exercises, speak with a licensed dietitian.

Prevent Injuries

Combining both cardiovascular and strength training can significantly reduce your risk of injury.

Muscle growth can become more balanced with the use of strength exercises. When you only concentrate on cardio, you could overlook other muscle groups, which might cause muscular imbalances. These imbalances can put stress on joints and raise the risk of sprains and rips, among other problems. Strength training is included in exercise to make sure all main muscle groups are used, which promotes a more balanced physique and lowers the chance of injuries brought on by muscular imbalances.

Joint stability is greatly influenced by strength training. The connective tissues around your joints get stronger as you gain muscle. With more stability, overuse injuries can be avoided, which are common during vigorous aerobic exercises like jogging. Stronger joints are less prone to tendonitis and ligament sprains, for example. For the stability of the entire body, a strong core is necessary. While some core muscles are used during cardiac workouts, core-specific exercises can further develop core strength.

Individual Considerations

- **Fitness Goals:** Your fitness objectives should dictate the balance between cardio and strength training. A bigger amount of your program should be devoted to cardio if you're trying to lose weight. Strength training, on the other hand, should take precedence if you want to put on muscle.

- **Time Restrictions:** Your workout balance is significantly influenced by your schedule. High-intensity interval training (HIIT), which mixes cardio and strength training into brief, intense sessions, is a good option if you only have a small amount of time to work.

- **Medical conditions:** The balance may need to be changed to suit the demands of people with certain medical conditions, such as joint or heart difficulties. To develop a customized strategy, speak with a qualified trainer or healthcare expert.

- **Enjoyment:** Ultimately, consistency is key. Choose activities you enjoy to ensure you stick with your fitness routine. Include extra swimming in your routine if you enjoy it.

Sample Weekly Workout Plan

Here is an example of a weekly exercise schedule to assist you in striking a balance between cardio and strength training:

1. Monday: 30 minutes of full-body strength training followed by 30 minutes of moderate-intensity cardio.

2. Tuesday: 20 minutes of HIIT, followed by 20 minutes of stretching.

3. Wednesday: Rest or light yoga for recovery.

4. Thursday: 30 minutes of cardio (jogging) + 30 minutes of strength training (focus on upper body).

5. Friday: 20 minutes of HIIT + 20 minutes of stretching.

6. Saturday: 45 minutes of cardio (cycling) + 30 minutes of strength training (focus on lower body).

7. Sunday: Rest or light yoga for recovery.

This is just one example, and you should adapt it to your preferences and goals.

In Conclusion

Instead of being considered as a competition, the discussion between cardio and strength training can be viewed as a collaboration. The proper ratio between the two depends on your unique requirements and goals. Both are essential components of a comprehensive fitness program. Combining strength and aerobic exercise can give you the best of both worlds in terms of a healthy heart, lean muscles, and overall well-being.

Tracking Progress and Staying Motivated

Setting realistic goals and measuring achievements

Finding the drive to exercise on a daily basis might be difficult in our fast-paced world. Setting specific objectives and recognizing the causes of demotivation, on the other hand, might be the key to keeping a consistent training regimen. In this section, we will discuss the significance of goal planning and the typical reasons why people lose the desire to exercise.

Goal Setting: The Foundation of a Successful Fitness Journey

Goal setting is the process of defining specific, achievable objectives that you aim to reach within a predetermined time frame. These goals work as a road map, directing your behaviors and efforts toward a desired conclusion. Goal setting in the context of fitness is determining what you want to achieve, whether it's decreasing weight, growing muscle, boosting endurance, or improving general health.

Short-term goals: These are smaller, more urgent goals that may generally be completed in a few weeks or months. After two months, you may, for example, raise your weekly running pace from one mile to three miles.

Long-term aims: These are more comprehensive, all-encompassing goals that will require more time and effort to fulfill. Long-term goals might include decreasing weight, running a marathon, or keeping to a regular training schedule for a year.

Understanding Demotivation

Here are some of the reasons why you feel demotivated

1. Lack of Visible Progress: One of the most common causes of demotivation is a sense of stagnation. It might be discouraging when you don't see obvious improvements in your physique or performance despite your efforts. To counter this, focus on small victories and trust the process.

2. Overwhelming Goals: Setting overly ambitious goals can lead to burnout and demotivation. When your goals seem too daunting, you may feel discouraged from even starting. Instead, break your objectives into manageable steps and gradually increase the intensity or difficulty.

3. Monotony: Doing the same workouts repeatedly can become monotonous and boring. To combat this, vary your exercise routine. Try new activities, classes, or workouts to keep things fresh and exciting.

4. External Pressures: Sometimes, external pressures, such as societal expectations or the desire to meet unrealistic beauty standards, can sap your motivation. It's crucial to exercise for your well-being and health rather than external validation.

5. Inadequate Rest: Overtraining and not allowing your body sufficient rest can lead to physical and mental fatigue. Adequate rest and recovery are integral parts of a successful fitness journey.

6. Lack of Accountability: Without accountability, it's easier to skip workouts. Consider finding a workout buddy or joining a fitness community to stay on track.

Why Do You Need to Set Goals?

Goals give you a strong feeling of direction. They outline your goals, allowing you to prioritize your efforts and keep focused on what's most essential. Without goals, your fitness journey can become aimless and less effective.

Goals serve as powerful motivators. It's simpler to stay devoted to your workouts when you have a clear goal in mind. The sense of achievement you get as you work toward your objectives may be quite motivating. Goals also offer a way to measure your progress objectively. You may monitor your progress and see how far you've come. This raises your confidence while also allowing you to make essential changes to your fitness program.

Having well-defined goals forces you to take responsibility for your actions. Setting a goal is a commitment to oneself that may boost your feeling of responsibility and discipline. Achieving your fitness objectives gives you a sense of success and fulfillment. It's an opportunity to celebrate your hard work and dedication, which can further fuel your motivation to set and reach new goals.

Goals can be changed as necessary. If you discover that a certain objective is either too difficult or not tough enough, you might change it to better suit your talents and desires.

Tips to stay motivated during exercise

Set Realistic Goals

Setting realistic objectives is the first step in remaining motivated throughout exercises. It's critical to be honest with yourself about where you are in terms of fitness and what you want to achieve. Setting unattainable objectives may lead to discontent and demotivation. Instead, divide your ambitions into smaller, more manageable benchmarks.

Make a Convenient Plan

It is vital to create a fitness plan, but it is much more crucial to make it convenient. Because life is busy, the more convenient your workout plan, the more likely you are to stick to it. Consider these tips:

- Schedule Wisely: Choose a workout time that aligns with your natural energy levels. If you're a morning person, a sunrise jog might be invigorating. Night owls might prefer an evening gym session.

- Location Matters: Pick a gym or workout spot that's close to your home or workplace. The less effort required to get there, the less room for excuses.

- Prepare Ahead: Lay out your workout clothing the night before, prepare your gym bag, and make a training schedule. Keep in mind that the more consistent you are, the faster you will notice benefits.

Find a Workout Buddy

Working out with a friend can make a world of difference in your motivation levels. Having a workout buddy creates a sense of accountability. You're less likely to bail on a workout if someone is waiting for you at the gym or the park. Plus, it can make exercise more enjoyable. You can chat, encourage each other, and celebrate your victories together.

Change Your Perspective

Sometimes, the key to staying motivated during workouts lies in shifting your perspective. Rather than seeing exercise as a duty, consider it an investment in your health and well-being. Consider these mindset shifts:

- Focus on How You Feel: Pay attention to the immediate benefits of exercise, such as increased energy and reduced stress. These short-term rewards can be motivating.

- Track Your Progress: To measure your progress, keep a workout log or use a fitness app. Every minor accomplishment should be celebrated. Seeing how far you've come might help you stay motivated.

- Variety is Spice: Don't be afraid to mix up your workouts. Trying new activities or classes can keep things interesting and prevent boredom.

Create a Positive Workout Environment

Creating a nice training atmosphere is one of the most effective strategies to keep motivated throughout workouts. Your training room should make you feel at ease, focused, and motivated.

Select a workout space that you genuinely enjoy being in. Whether it's a gym, your living room, or the great outdoors, make sure it suits your preferences and needs. Add elements that inspire and motivate you. Hang up motivational quotes, and posters of your fitness role models, or simply play music that gets you pumped up. A clutter-free workout area can help you stay focused. Arrange your equipment neatly, ensuring easy access and a clean, inviting atmosphere.

Schedule a Regular Workout Time

Establishing a consistent workout schedule is another key to maintaining motivation. When you stick to a regular workout schedule, it becomes an unavoidable part of your daily or weekly schedule. Decide how many days a week you can devote to working out. Be honest with yourself to avoid overcommitting and feeling discouraged.

Knowing what you'll do during each workout session adds structure to your routine. It also aids in the prevention of aimlessness, which can lead to demotivation. Try to exercise at the same time every day or week. Consistency strengthens the habit, making you less likely to skip exercises due to a lack of enthusiasm.

Reward Yourself

Rewarding yourself for reaching fitness milestones can be a powerful motivator. It provides positive reinforcement and makes your fitness journey more enjoyable. Break your long-term fitness goals into smaller, achievable milestones. For example, if your ultimate goal is to run a marathon, set milestones for completing certain distances or improving your time in shorter races. When you achieve a milestone, reward yourself with something that genuinely excites you. It could be a spa day, a new workout outfit, or a guilt-free treat meal. Maintain a fitness notebook to keep track of your improvement. Keeping track of your accomplishments may be quite motivating, especially when you look back and realize how far you've come.

Listen to Your Body

Learning to listen to your body is one of the most important components of keeping motivated throughout exercises. While pushing yourself to develop is crucial, it's also necessary to know when your body needs a rest. Excessive effort might result in burnout and demotivation. Watch for indicators of weariness, soreness, or discomfort and alter your workout intensity accordingly. Fitness progress is a journey, and it's critical to respect your body's boundaries to avoid injuries and stay motivated.

Create a Fun Playlist

Music has a remarkable influence on our mood and motivation. Curate a workout playlist filled with your favorite upbeat songs. Music can provide the energy and enthusiasm needed to power through your workouts. Experiment with different genres and tempos to keep things fresh. The right music can make even the most challenging workouts feel more enjoyable, helping you stay engaged and motivated.

Adjust Your Tempo

Variety is the spice of life, and your exercises are no exception. Doing the same thing every day might lead to boredom and demotivation. To combat this, change the pace of your workouts regularly. Incorporate different exercises, try new fitness classes, or explore outdoor activities like hiking or cycling. Mixing things up not only keeps your workouts interesting but also challenges your body in different ways, promoting continuous progress.

Take Breaks Mid-Workout

Taking small breaks throughout your training might actually enhance motivation, which may seem paradoxical. These breaks help you to rehydrate, regain your breath, and refocus your thoughts. Structured rest intervals can also improve your performance during high-intensity workouts. Consider incorporating interval training, where you alternate between intense exercises and brief rest periods. This approach not only keeps motivation high but can also lead to significant fitness gains.

Track Your Progress

Visible improvement in your fitness quest may be a great motivation. Keep a workout notebook to track your progress, such as the number of reps, sets, or time spent working out. Take regular measures of your body, such as your weight, body fat percentage, and body dimensions. Tracking these metrics provides a visual representation of your progress, which can be incredibly motivating. Celebrate your milestones, no matter how small they may seem, as they signify your dedication and hard work paying off.

Read Workout Quotes

Drawing inspiration from fitness quotes is one of the easiest yet most effective methods to keep motivated throughout workouts. These pearls of wisdom are more than simply catchy words; they may also serve as a tremendous source of motivation. When you're about to give up or struggle through a difficult workout, read a motivating quotation to remember why you started in the first place.

Overcome Common Challenges

Obstacles are an unavoidable element of every fitness program. Identifying and addressing these challenges head-on can help you stay motivated. Busy schedules often top the list of reasons people skip workouts. To overcome this obstacle, plan your exercises like any other appointment. Make them non-negotiable and top priority.

When you reach a plateau and see no improvement, it might be discouraging. To break through these plateaus, change up your regimen, try new workouts, or seek advice from a fitness specialist. We've all had days when we're too exhausted to exercise. On such days, attempt a shorter, less difficult workout or participate in an activity that you truly like.

Conclusion

Setting specific, realistic, time-bound, and quantifiable goals provides concentration and motivation. Understanding the root reasons for demotivation and taking action to address them can also assist you in staying on track. Remember that staying motivated is an adventure in and of itself and that with the right mindset and strategies, you can achieve your fitness goals and stick to a steady training regimen.

Mindful Ageing Through Strength Training

Exploring the concept of aging mindfully and how strength training can support it

---

As we journey through life, one inevitability we all face is the process of aging. It's an undeniable fact, a natural course of life. But how we age and the quality of life we lead as we grow older can greatly depend on our approach to this phenomenon. Enter mindful aging, a concept that encourages us to embrace the passing years with grace and wisdom, while ensuring our bodies and minds remain vibrant and active. In this article, we'll explore what mindful aging entails and delve into how strength training can play a pivotal role in this transformative journey.

What is Mindful Aging?

Mindful aging is about extending years of our lives rather than simply years to our lives. Mindful aging encompasses a holistic perspective on getting older, emphasizing the importance of self-awareness and engaging in proactive endeavors that safeguard our mental, emotional, and physical well-being. In its essence, it involves embracing the wisdom that accompanies the march of time, tending to the needs of our bodies and minds, and seeking happiness and fulfillment throughout every stage of life.

How Does Aging Impact Our Bodies?

The progressive loss of muscular mass is perhaps one of the first signs of aging. This phenomenon, scientifically referred to as sarcopenia, initiates its subtle journey around the age of 30 and picks up pace as we traverse our 40s and venture into our 50s.

Sarcopenia can bring about a decrease in strength and mobility, increasing the risk of falls. Aging also ushers in a decrease in bone density, rendering our bones more susceptible to fractures. This is when conditions like osteoporosis become more prevalent, posing a substantial health concern.

With age, joint mobility tends to decrease, leading to stiffness and discomfort. Take arthritis, for instance. It tends to worsen with time, producing chronic discomfort and impeding our daily activities. Growing older can also have an impact on our cognitive abilities.

Then there's the problem with metabolism. It progressively diminishes, making weight gain simpler and maintaining a healthy shape more challenging. Hormonal changes, such as increasing estrogen and testosterone levels, can also cause mental and physical changes.

Although these adjustments are unavoidable as we become older, the theory of mindful aging urges us to be proactive in dealing with them. This is when the value of strength training becomes clear.

The Importance of Strength Training as We Age

When pondering the art of aging gracefully, the thought of strength training might not immediately spring to mind. Often associated with the younger generation or athletes, it's a facet of fitness that deserves our attention as we journey through the golden years. Strength training, surprisingly, boasts a myriad of benefits for individuals on the path of aging, which include:

1. Immune System Enhancement

Our immune systems decrease as we age, making us more prone to infections and diseases. This is where strength training may help significantly. Regular strength training workouts can help strengthen our immune systems. When we commit to resistance training, something fascinating happens within our bodies. They respond by ramping up the production of those trusty white blood cells, the foot soldiers in our immune system's army, ready to fend off infections and illnesses. Strengthening our immune system through resistance training can truly bolster our health and vitality as we gracefully navigate the journey of aging.

2. Improved Sleep

Quality sleep becomes increasingly elusive for many as they age. SS strength training offers an additional boon - it can assist in combating insomnia. The magic behind this lies in the release of endorphins when we engage in exercise, especially the kind that involves strength training. These endorphins don't just work wonders for our mood; they also play a role in promoting restful sleep. Furthermore, the physical weariness caused by strength exercise might contribute to a deeper and more peaceful sleep. Adequate sleep is essential for general well-being, and strength training can help us sleep better as we age.

3. Decreased Blood Pressure

Elevated blood pressure, often known as hypertension, is a common worry, particularly among the elderly, and it can possibly lead to serious health consequences. Consistent participation in strength training exercises can bring about remarkable improvements in the flexibility and overall health of our blood vessels, thereby facilitating smoother blood circulation. Consequently, this leads to a reduced burden on the heart and a subsequent drop in blood pressure. Engaging in regular physical activity holds significant promise in not only managing but also preventing hypertension.

4. Improved Chronic Pain

Chronic pain is a persistent companion for many seniors, affecting their daily lives and overall well-being. Strength training offers a path towards pain relief. Strength training can help with chronic pain problems like arthritis and lower back pain by strengthening the muscles around joints and increasing overall musculoskeletal health. It also improves flexibility and balance, lowering the chance of falls and related accidents, which frequently aggravate chronic pain.

5. Embracing Change

One of the fundamental steps towards mindful aging involves wholeheartedly embracing the natural transformations that accompany the passage of time. Strength training serves as a guiding light towards this acceptance, promoting a profound sense of body consciousness. Through engaging in strength-based exercises, a profound connection with your body's capabilities and constraints emerges. This heightened awareness becomes the catalyst for acceptance, enabling you to truly admire your body for its unique state at any given point in your life. Rather than fixating on what you might have relinquished over the years, you start to cherish what can be accomplished through consistent dedication.

6. Cultivating Resilience

Aging unfurls a journey teeming with both moments of joy and trials. The process of building physical strength through regular training not only bolsters your body's resiliency but also nurtures an enduring mental fortitude. The dedication and resolve demanded by consistent strength training seamlessly translate into an unwavering sense of mental strength. It's here that you come to realize that setbacks are an inherent facet of the journey, and with persistence and patience, you possess the capacity to surmount them. This newfound resilience ripples into other dimensions of your life, providing you with the tools to gracefully navigate the ebb and flow of aging's challenges.

7. A Gentle Heart

Compassion towards oneself stands as a pillar of mindful aging. Strength training, in its essence, provides a unique platform for fostering self-compassion. It permits you to set goals that are within reach and to commemorate every small triumph along your journey. Through recognition of your own progress and an embrace of self-compassion, you lay the foundation for a positive rapport with your body, an indispensable facet of a gratifying aging process. Engaging in regular physical activity, including strength training, releases endorphins, promoting a positive mood and reducing stress. This compassionate outlook reaches beyond just physical well-being, extending its influence on how you connect with others and the world that surrounds you.

8. Heightened Awareness

Mindful aging necessitates a heightened awareness of both your physical and emotional states. Strength training plays a pivotal role in nurturing this awareness by compelling you to be fully present in each moment. Every repetition, every breath, beckons your undivided attention. This intensified mindfulness not only elevates the efficacy of your training but spills into your everyday life. You gradually attune yourself to the unique needs of your body, thus empowering you to make more informed choices concerning your overall health and holistic well-being.

9. Building Strong Bones

As we gracefully traverse the path of aging, there's an aspect that sometimes escapes our notice but merits our full consideration: the well-being of our bones. As time unfurls its tapestry, our bone density often experiences a decline, rendering us more vulnerable to fractures and the ominous presence of osteoporosis. Nevertheless, there exists a formidable companion in our arsenal - the practice of strength training. This isn't merely about the act of lifting weights; it entails engaging in weight-bearing exercises like squats, deadlifts, and bench presses. These activities transcend the mere deceleration of bone density loss; they possess the potential to fortify it. In simpler terms, they help you maintain that confident and upright posture well into your golden years.

10. Manage Your Weight

Aging has its own set of difficulties, notably in terms of weight control. This uphill battle is fueled by shifts in metabolism and activity levels. Nevertheless, maintaining an optimal weight is vital for overall well-being. Strength training steps into the arena as a formidable contender. By increasing muscle mass, it gives your resting metabolic rate a nudge upwards.

11. Having a Good Time

This is where strength training takes center stage in enhancing your overall quality of life. It's the key to unlocking greater flexibility and balance, thus diminishing the risk of unfortunate tumbles and injuries. This newfound physical resilience doesn't just keep you on your feet; it also enables you to maintain your independence, letting you savor the activities you hold dear for a longer stretch. What's more, the act of strength training releases those delightful endorphins – the body's natural mood enhancers – thereby diminishing the shadow of depression and uplifting your mental and emotional well-being.

12. Exercising the Mind

The advantages of strength training don't stop at the physical realm; they extend their reach into cognitive enhancement. As we journey through the chapters of life, cognitive decline can cast a long shadow. Yet, research has unveiled a rather intriguing connection between regular strength training and the preservation of mental acuity. It triggers the release of brain-derived neurotrophic factor, a fascinating protein that plays a crucial role in supporting brain well-being. The result is Sharper thinking skills, a fortified memory, and the potential to thwart the onset of daunting neurodegenerative ailments like Alzheimer's.

13. Manage Chronic Conditions

Aging gracefully often entails dealing with a slew of persistent health issues that can substantially affect our daily lives. Conditions like arthritis, osteoporosis, and diabetes frequently accompany the aging process, making routine activities challenging and occasionally painful.

Strength training has, through research and experience, proven to be a valuable ally in managing chronic conditions. Strength training can alleviate the discomfort that conditions like arthritis bring, courtesy of the enhanced support and stability offered by stronger muscles around affected joints.

Taking a mindful approach to strength training enables individuals to tailor their workouts to their specific requirements, steadily bolstering strength and resilience while minimizing any potential aggravation of chronic conditions. It's imperative, though, to engage in a dialogue with a healthcare expert or fitness professional to craft a well-rounded and secure strength training regimen that aligns with your unique circumstances.

14. Preserving Muscle Mass

Perhaps one of the most conspicuous transformations that our bodies undergo as we age is the gradual diminishment of muscle mass, a phenomenon referred to as sarcopenia. This decline in muscle isn't merely superficial; it has a tangible impact on our functional abilities. However, the inclusion of strength training emerges as a formidable ally in the quest to retain muscle mass and function as the years go by.

Strength training wages a relentless battle against muscle loss by prompting muscle growth and maintenance. This occurs through a process known as muscle hypertrophy, where individual muscle fibers enlarge. Mindful aging through strength training involves a gradual and progressive approach, emphasizing proper form and technique to prevent injury. It's advisable to seek guidance from a qualified trainer to design a personalized workout plan that suits your age and fitness level.

Conclusion

In conclusion, mindful aging is a philosophy that encourages us to approach the aging process with intention and awareness. While changes to our bodies and thoughts are unavoidable as we age, we do have the ability to affect how we age. Strength training is an important tool in our journey, as it helps us preserve physical vitality and general well-being while we calmly accept the passing of time. We may live our latter years with vigor, knowledge, and a love for life that defies age by taking a conscious approach to aging and adding strength training into our lives.

Senior Success Stories in Strength Training

Sharing real-life stories of seniors who have benefited from incorporating strength training into their lives

---

Step into a world of determination, growth, and achievement with us! We're excited to bring you the genuine stories of older adults who have reaped the incredible benefits of making strength training an integral part of their daily routines in this section. These are stories of knowledge, tenacity, and a spirit that transcends age prejudices.

Strength training isn't just for the young and the restless. It's a transformative practice that knows no age boundaries. Our senior success stories serve as a testament to the fact that you can build strength, improve mobility, and experience a vibrant, fulfilling life well into your golden years.

Prepare to be inspired as we delve into the lives of these incredible individuals who've discovered newfound vigor through strength training. Their journeys will touch your heart and perhaps even motivate you to embark on your own path to a healthier, stronger you.

Transformation # 1:

One day, Kevin found himself in a pickle when he needed to get up from the floor but couldn't. Kevin's wife thought it was time for a change after witnessing her husband's misery and enrolled him in a fitness program. Fast forward nine months, and Kevin can now easily rise from the floor, a feat he once found challenging.

When Kevin first began his fitness journey under the guidance of a dedicated trainer, he could barely stand up from a chair more than a few times. But today, he confidently performs multiple sets of weighted squats with grace. Thanks to a tailored exercise regimen, Kevin has experienced a reduction in lower body swelling, significant weight loss, and an increase in muscle tone.

Kevin's flexibility, overall strength, endurance, and balance have all undergone remarkable improvements. In the past, he often experienced muscle cramps during stretching due to tight muscles. Now, those cramps are a thing of the past, and Kevin feels more agile than ever. His cardiovascular endurance has seen a substantial boost, allowing him to comfortably extend his treadmill walks by an extra 5-7 minutes compared to just a few months ago. While achieving better balance remains a goal for Kevin, he's already made progress. He could only keep an upright position (one foot in front of the other) for a few seconds at first, but he can now hold it for around 30 seconds. He's also learned more difficult moves like lunges, which demand a lot of balance. Kevin has also enhanced his general strength and is now lifting greater weights than he has in a long time.

Perhaps one of the most rewarding achievements is Kevin's newfound perspective on exercise. He occasionally reveals after a session how amazing he feels and how much he appreciates the experience.

Kevin says "It's well worth the effort. Getting into shape takes time, but it's truly rewarding. My clothes fit better, and I feel better. I've discovered muscles I had forgotten about,".

Transformation # 2:

During a routine exam at a local clinic for a completely unrelated health issue, I received some surprising news: I had severe osteoporosis. It caught me off guard, so I decided to seek a second opinion. I proceeded to another institution for another bone density test, and the findings confirmed my earlier diagnosis.

Coincidentally, while grappling with this news, I happened to catch a radio report discussing some intriguing research that piqued my interest. I contacted the physical therapists at a local rehabilitation clinic because I was intrigued by the possible applicability of this study to my situation. Thankfully they were eager to work with me on designing a customized fitness routine based on the study's findings.

I diligently adhered to this program, which consisted of weight lifting and regular walks. Most days, I continue my weightlifting routine at home, sparing me the need to visit the gym multiple times a week.

I'm absolutely thrilled to share that my most recent bone density scan revealed improvements. While my physician has consistently attributed this progress to my treatment, I am firmly convinced that the exercise program I followed played a substantial role in transforming my bone density from a severe osteoporosis diagnosis to a less severe case known as osteopenia. Though I'm not a statistician, the concept of young individuals shifting from two standard deviations below the average to 85% of the projected peak bone density seems quite excellent to me.

Warm regards,

Eleanor

Transformation # 3:

For over five decades now, Noah Anderson has been on a remarkable journey, determined to challenge the inevitable impact of aging by embracing the art of weightlifting. Noah began weightlifting at the youthful age of 17 in 1944, with the distinct purpose of cultivating his well-being. "If it wasn't a genuine passion," Noah says with a smile, "I wouldn't have committed to it for a whopping 56 years." At the age of 72, Noah is still a strong supporter of the healthy lifestyle he has developed over the years. His wife of 52 years has also joined him in their fitness journey for the past eight years.

However, the advantages of regular exercise extend beyond physical health for Noah. He believes that remaining physically active has a positive impact on one's mental health. According to him, exercising has the ability to raise your self-esteem and overall confidence. He also attests to how it improves interpersonal skills by instilling confidence.

In his younger years, Noah was constantly pushing his limits to lift more weight and achieve new milestones. However, he now follows a well-established routine that suits his current needs. His regimen includes walking, using a stationary bike, and a carefully designed weightlifting routine. Noah dedicates four to five days a week to workouts, with each session lasting between 30 to 60 minutes. He views his exercise routine as a way to maintain his overall health.

In addition to maintaining his own fitness, Noah has a strong desire to connect with other seniors in his community. He firmly holds the belief that it's never too late to start a fitness journey. Noah advises anyone contemplating a new exercise regimen to have a chat with their healthcare provider beforehand.

Noah's aspiration is to host seminars for seniors, enlightening them about the myriad benefits of weight training. Although many senior citizens may have concerns about potential injuries, Noah emphasizes the numerous advantages of weightlifting. He points out some significant health advantages too, including warding off issues such as osteoporosis, adult-onset diabetes, and colon cancer. Plus, pumping iron plays a role in helping you achieve a more toned physique and curbing excess weight. Noah also asserts that it can be instrumental in alleviating mental depression while enhancing overall strength and flexibility.

This sprightly senior citizen is determined to continue his fitness journey for as long as possible. "I've maintained my mental alertness, thanks to weight training and exercise," Noah concludes with a smile.

Transformation # 4:

Coping with the loss of a loved one and juggling a demanding online teaching job took a toll on Sarah's physical well-being. Her posture slumped, and she struggled to ascend the stairs, needing to grasp the railing with both hands for support.

Between January and April, Sarah and her trainer collaborated on improving her leg strength, spinal flexibility, mobility, and balance. She now effortlessly climbs stairs, often performing weighted exercises on them without relying on handrails.

Her trainer said "During our initial assessment, we measured her balance, and the progress has been remarkable. Her ability to stand in tandem (one foot in front of the other) has increased from 10 seconds to over 2 minutes! Sarah's constant quest for greater challenges is truly inspiring; her motivation to always improve drives her forward."

Sarah's perspective:

"It's hard to find the words to express my gratitude for my trainer's incredible help in my journey to regain my mobility and independence after a significant setback."

Conclusion

As we draw the curtain on these remarkable senior success stories, we hope you've been as inspired as we have by the indomitable spirit of these individuals. Strength training has been shown over and again to be a timeless elixir for a strong, active, and satisfying existence.

We encourage you to take these stories to heart as a wellspring of motivation, regardless of where you find yourself on your personal journey. Always remember, it's never too late to embark on or persist in your pursuit of strength, vitality, and a richly rewarding life. Whether you're a senior in search of inspiration or someone who's reached their senior years, we trust these narratives will underscore the idea that age is no barrier to strength, and your most fulfilling days might still be on the horizon. Embrace the transformative potential of strength training and allow your own tale of success to gradually unfold.

Illustrated Guide of Strength and Balance Exercises for Seniors

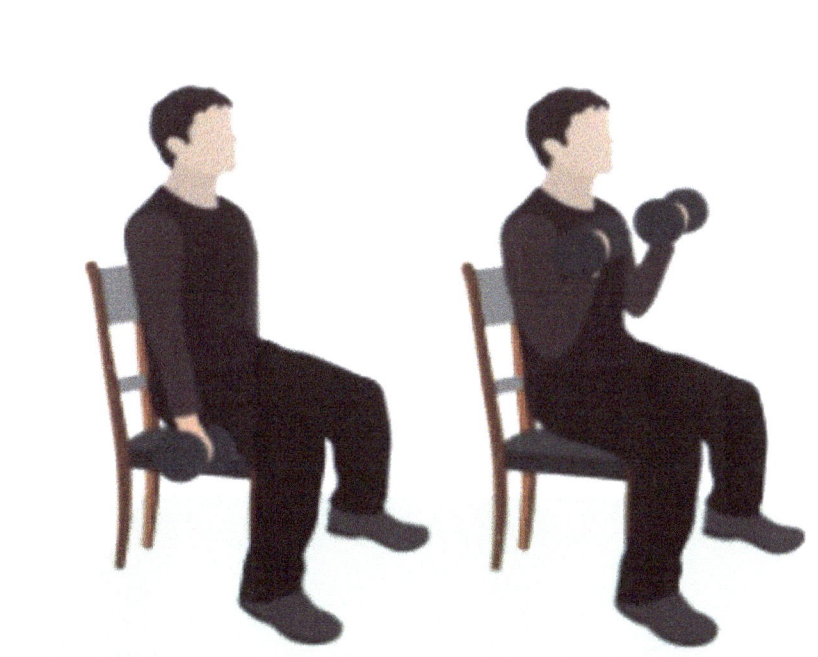

Chair Bicep Curls

Sit on the chair, hold a dumbbell in each hand, and curl the weights up towards your shoulders.

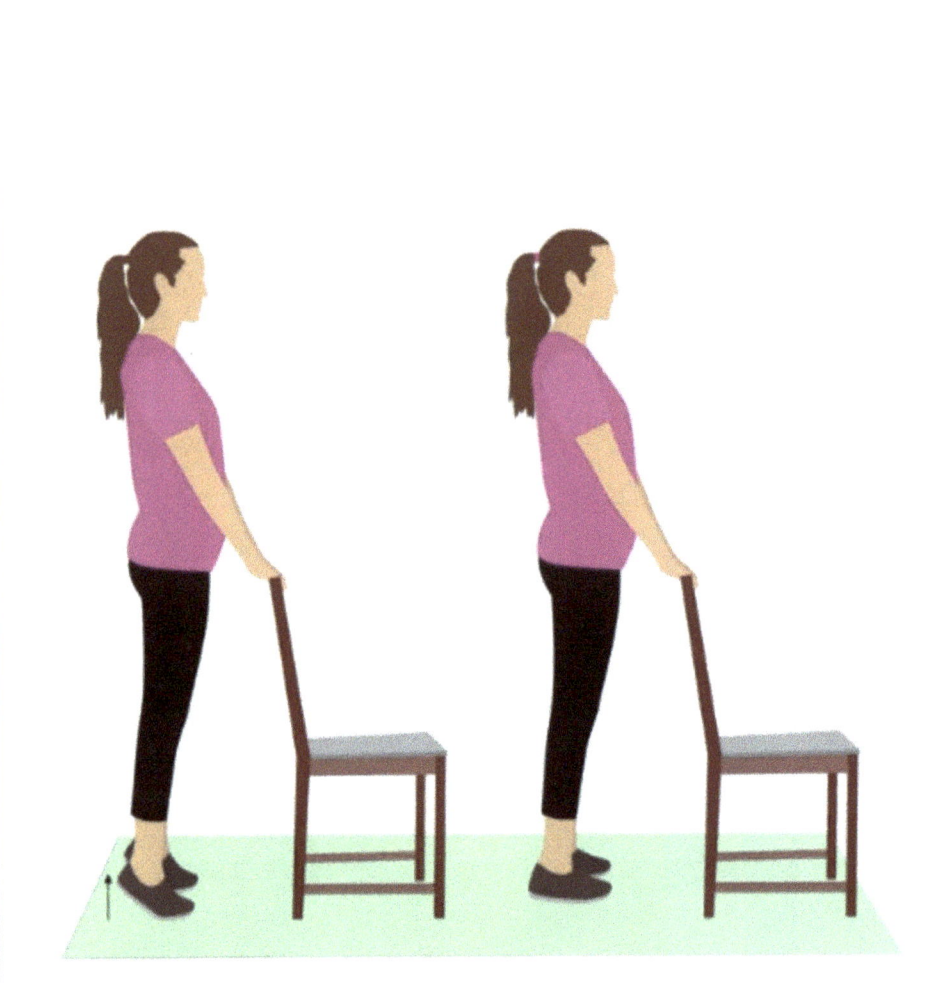

Chair Calf Raises

Stand behind the chair, rise onto tiptoes, then lower your heels.

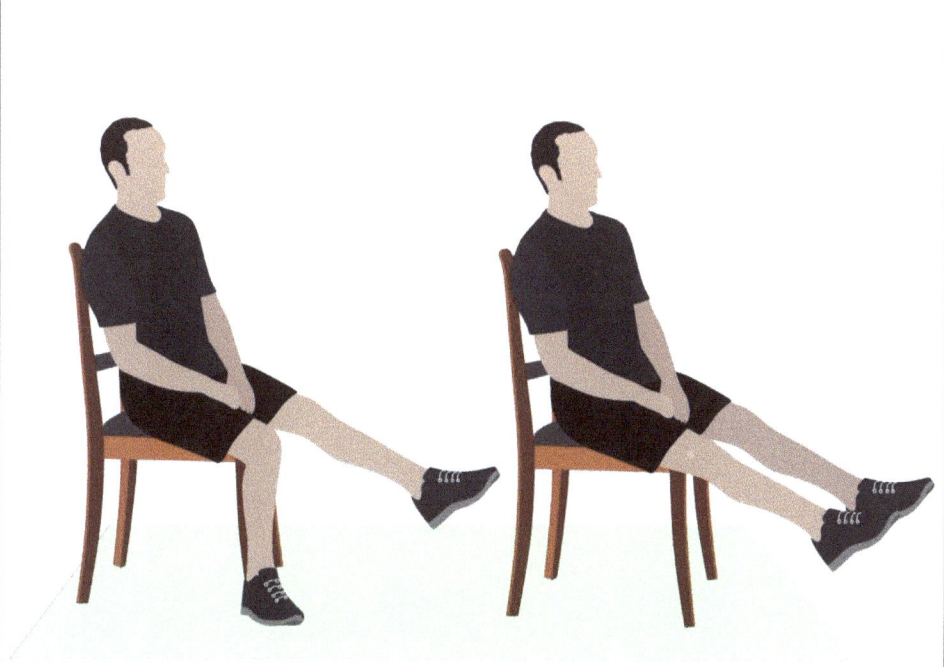

Chair Hamstring Curls

Sit on the chair, slide your feet back and forth, bending and straightening your knees.

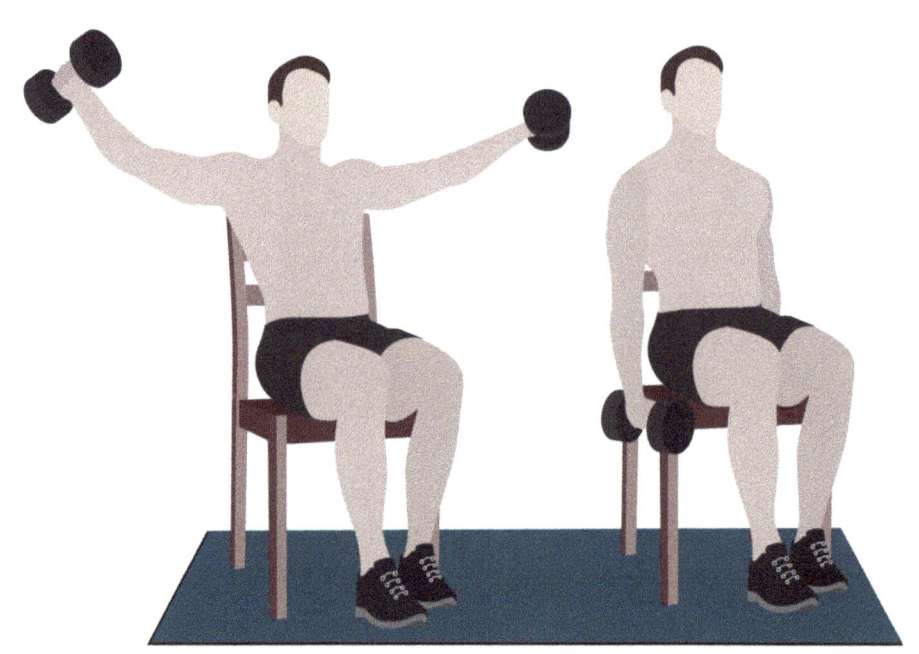

Chair Lateral Raises

Sit on the chair, hold a dumbbell in each hand at your sides, then lift them out to shoulder height.

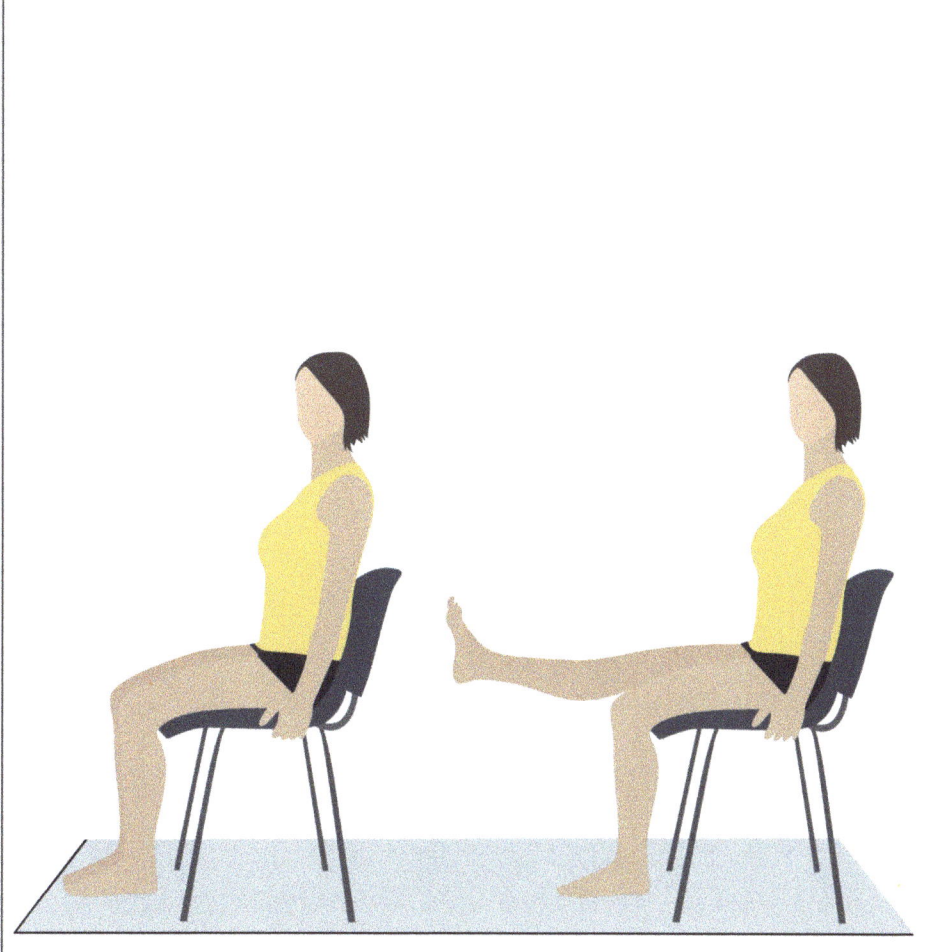

Chair Leg Extensions

Sit on the chair, extend one leg straight out, hold briefly, then lower it.

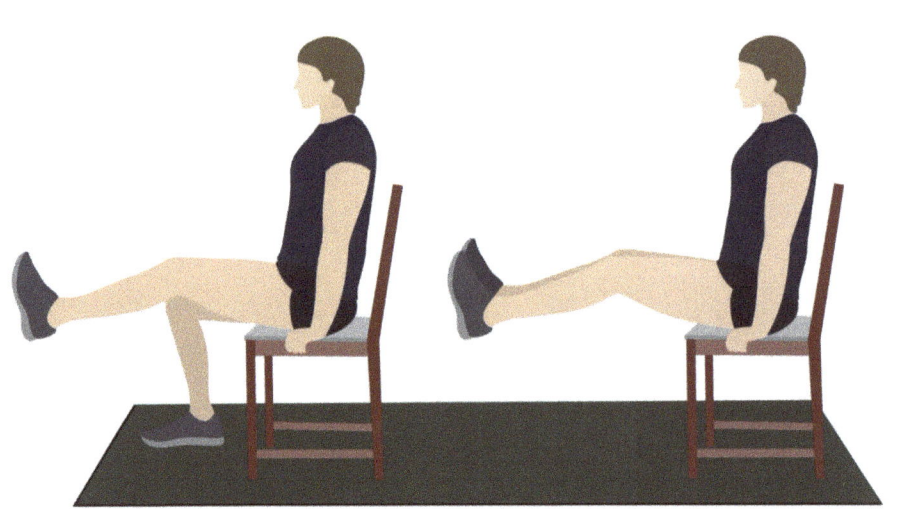

Chair Leg Raises

Sit on the chair, extend one leg straight out and hold briefly, then lower it back down. alternate legs.

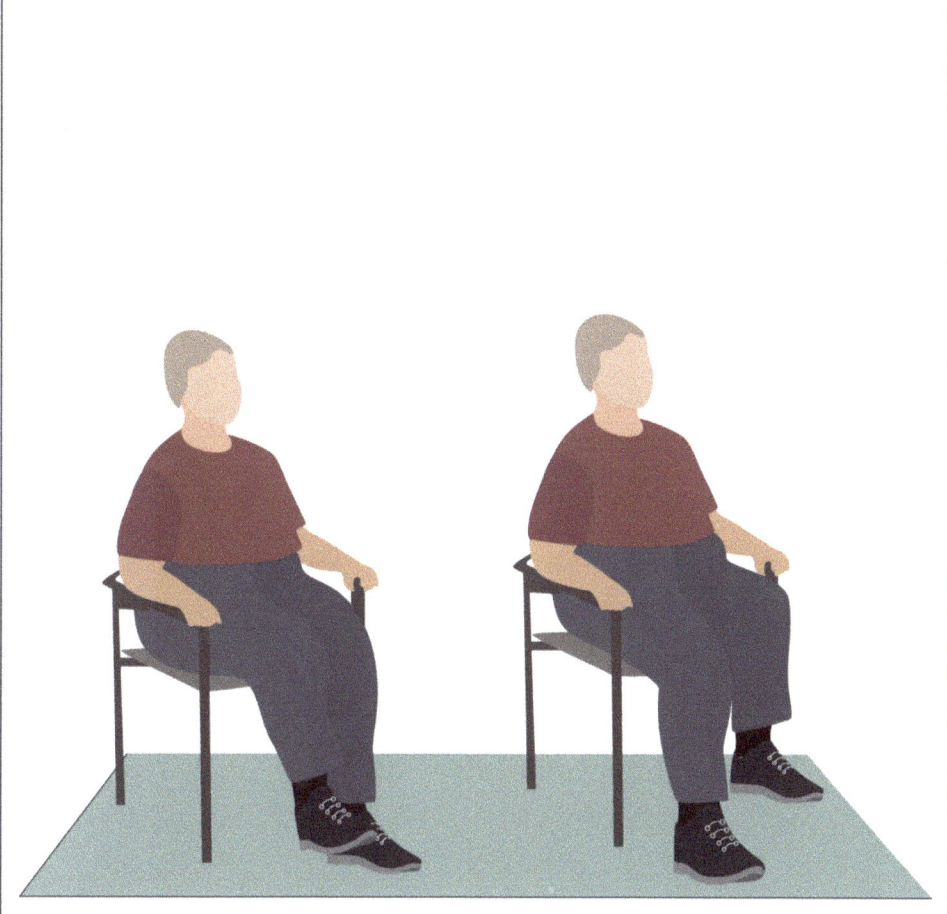

Chair Marching

Sit on chair with feet flat on the floor. Lift one knee at a time, as if you were marching in place.

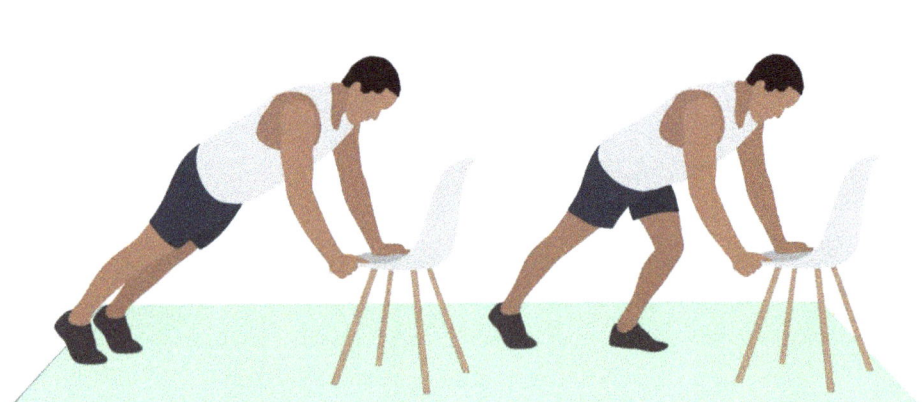

Chair Mountain Climbers

Assume a push up position with your hands on the seat of the chair, and alternate bringing your knees towards your chest.

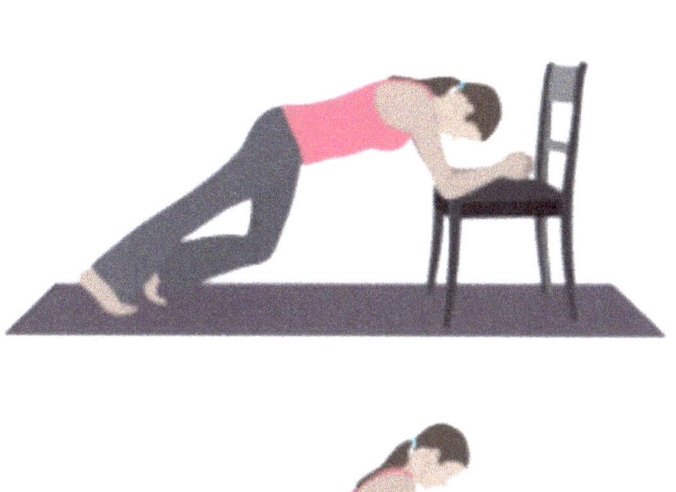

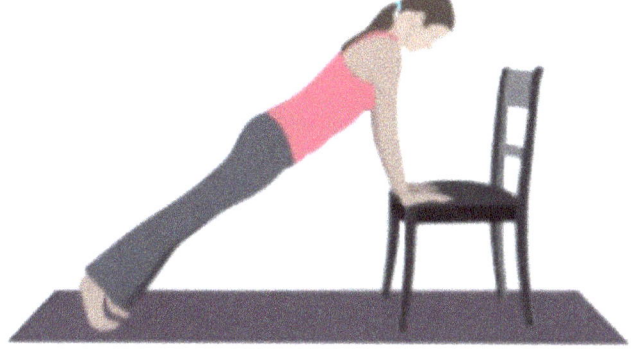

Chair Plank

Place your hands on the seat of the chair and extend your legs behind you, holding a plank position.

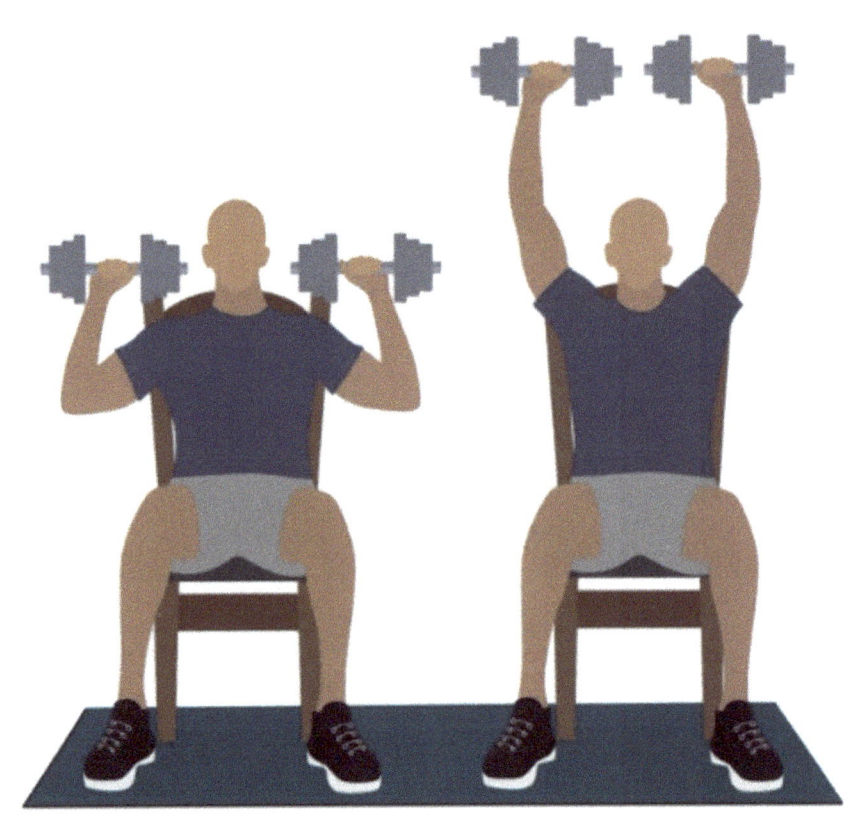

Chair Shoulder Press

Sit on the chair, hold a dumbbell in each hand at shoulder height, then press them upwards.

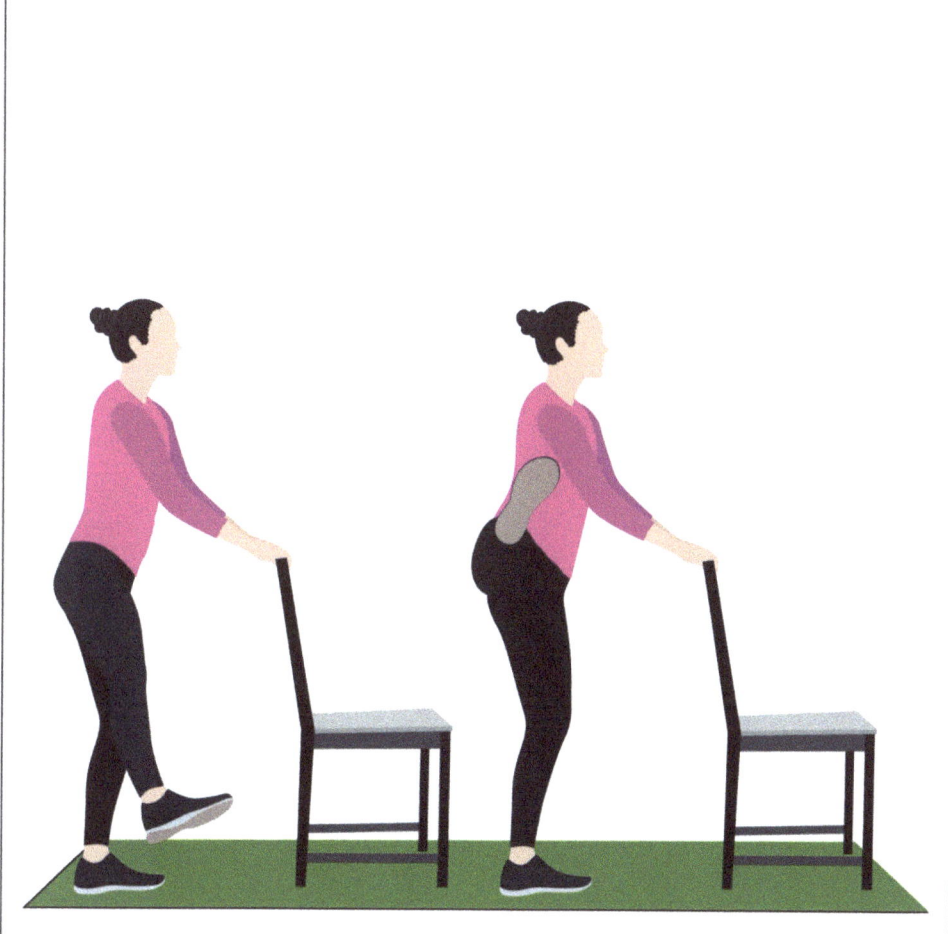

Chair Side Leg Raises

Stand on the back of chair, lift one leg out to the side, then lower it back down, alternate legs.

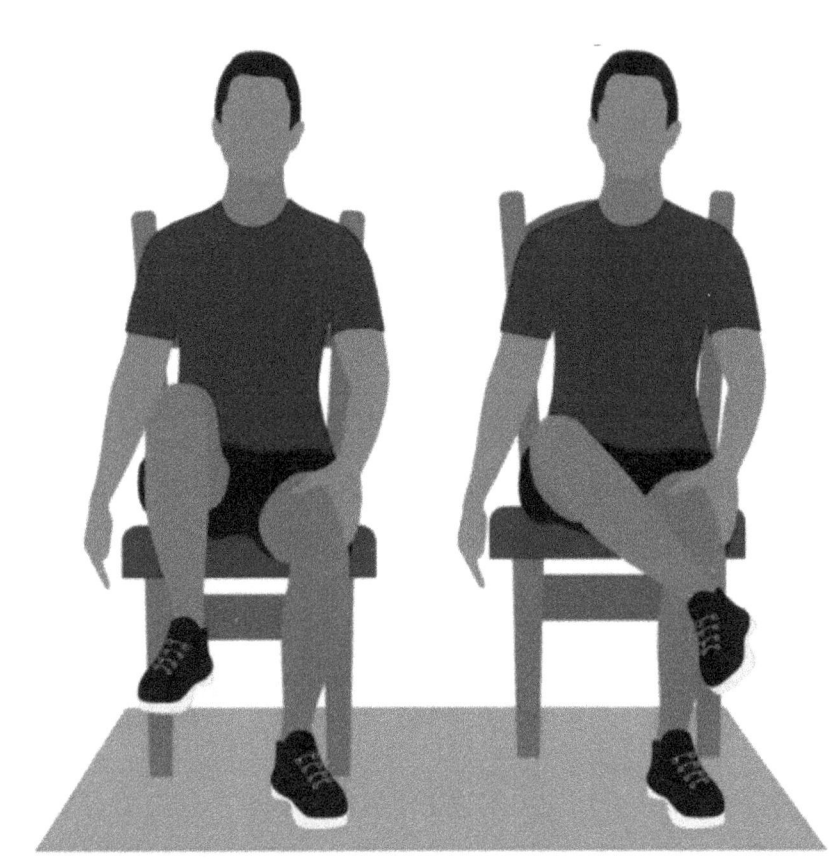

Chair Single Knee Lifts

Sit on a chair, lift one knee towards your chest, then lower it back down. Alternate between knees for single knee lifts.

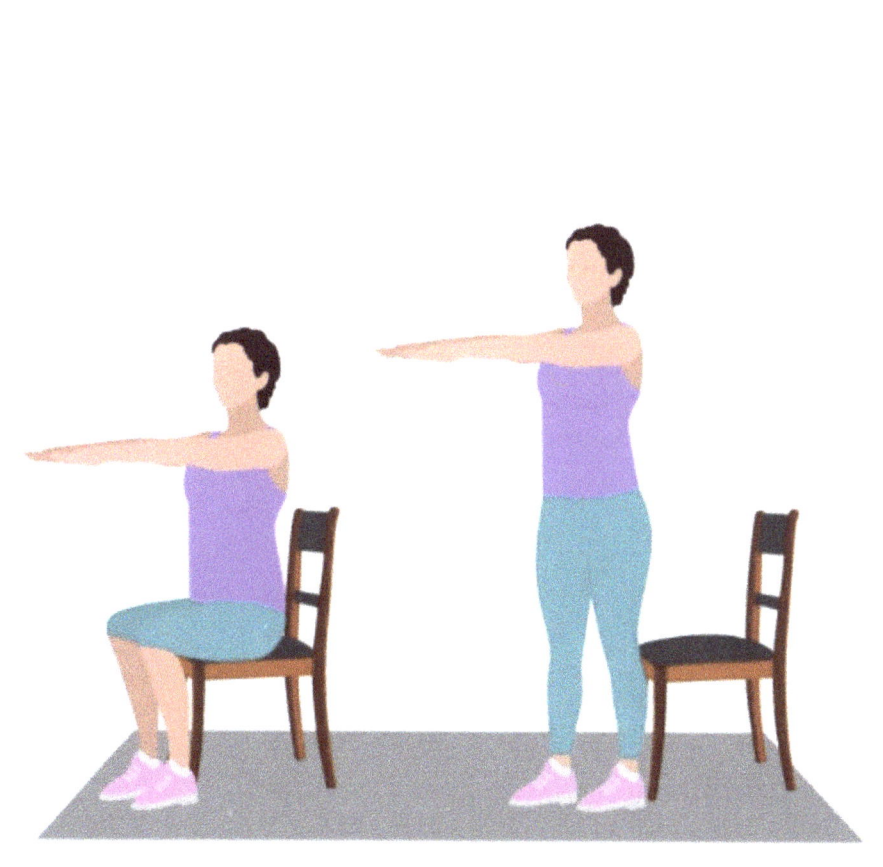

Chair Squats with Hand Raise

Perform chair squats, raising your hands as you lower your body as if sitting, and return to a standing position.

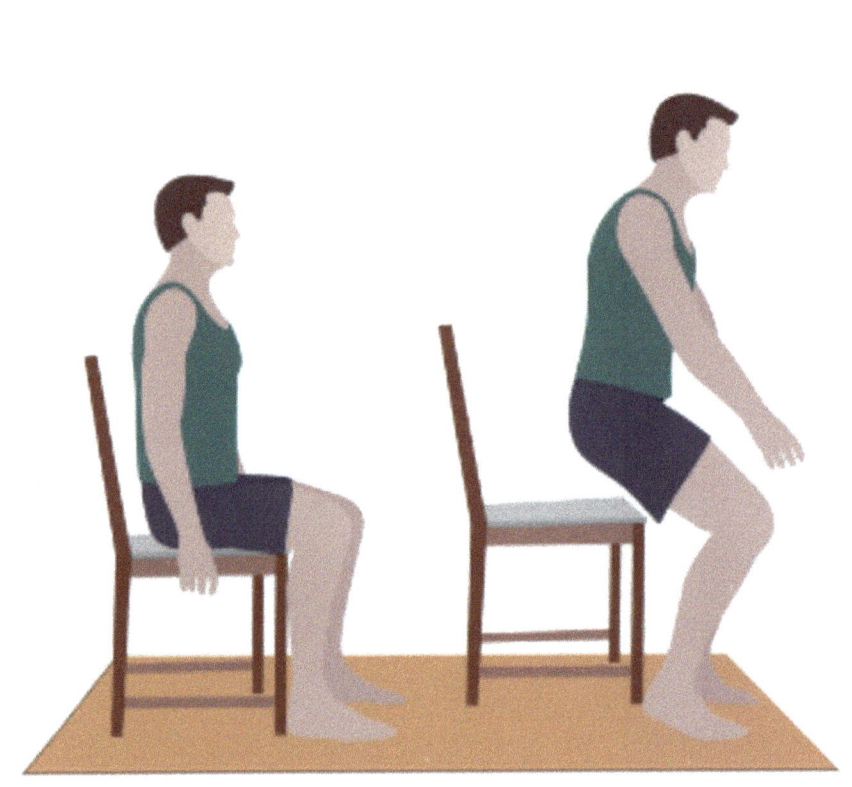

Chair Squats

Stand in front of the chair, lower your body as if sitting, then return to a standing position.

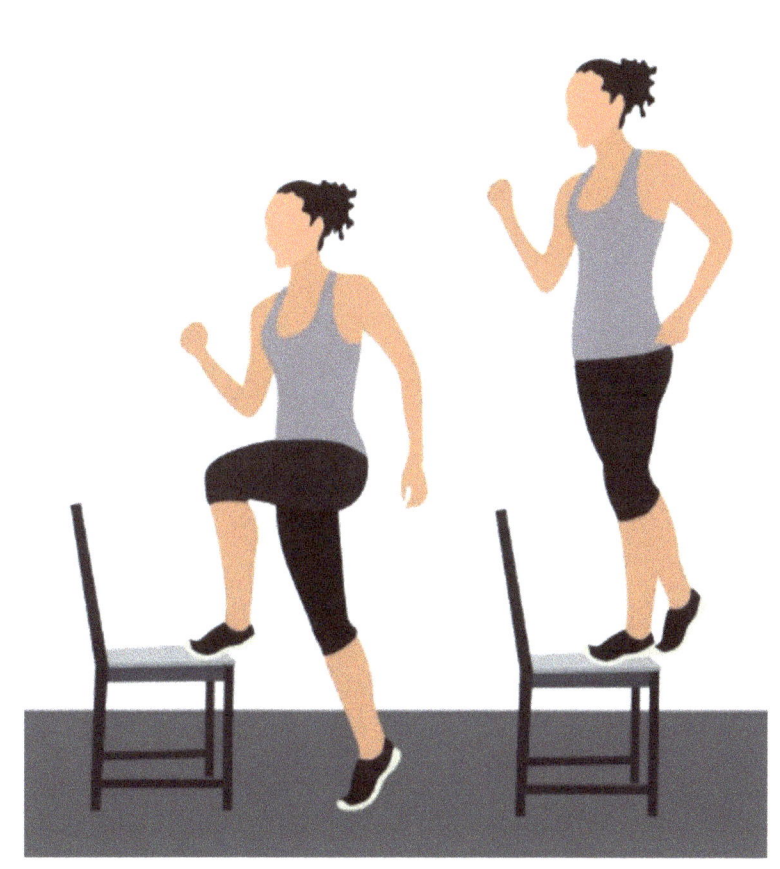

Chair Step-ups

Stand in front of the chair, step one foot onto the seat, then step back down, alternate legs.

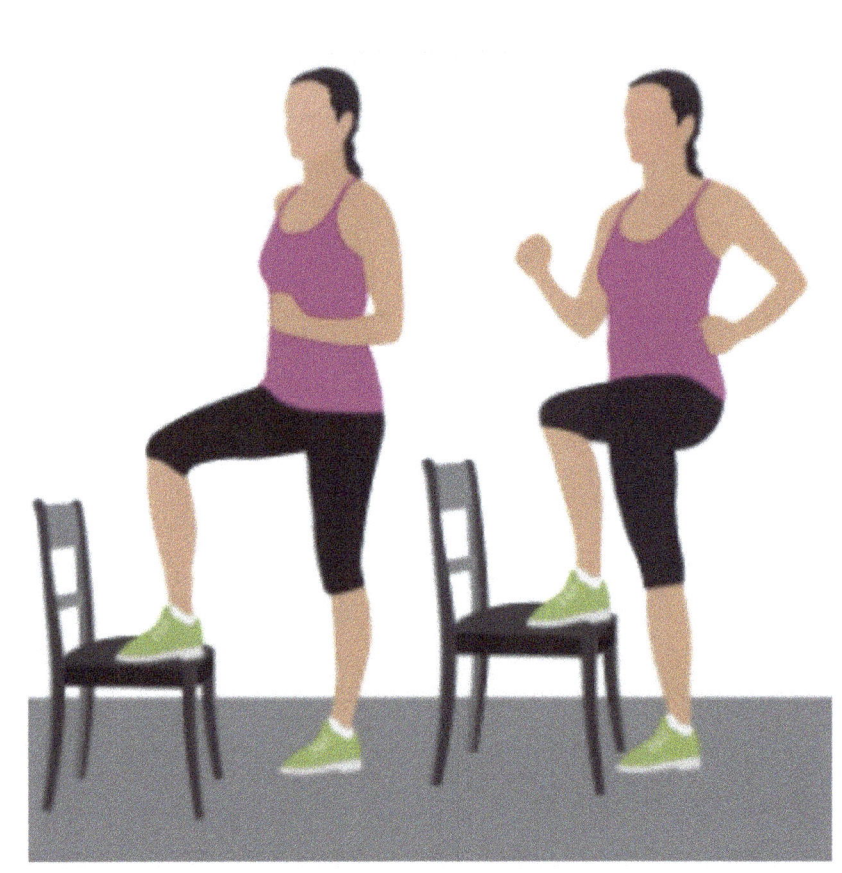

Chair Step-ups

Stand in front of the chair, step one foot onto the seat, then step back down, alternate legs.

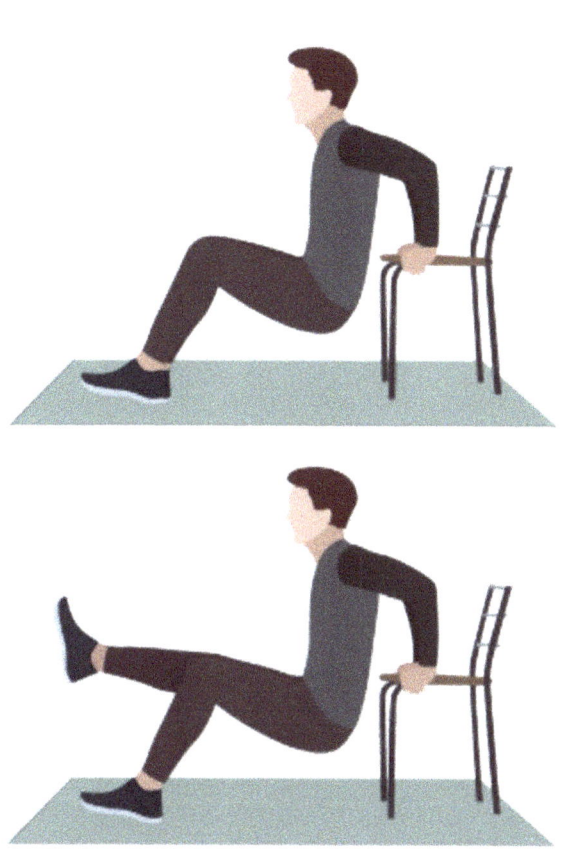

Chair Triceps Extensions

Sit on the chair, grasp the front edges, extend arms straight, then bent at the elbows to lower your body and straighten them again.

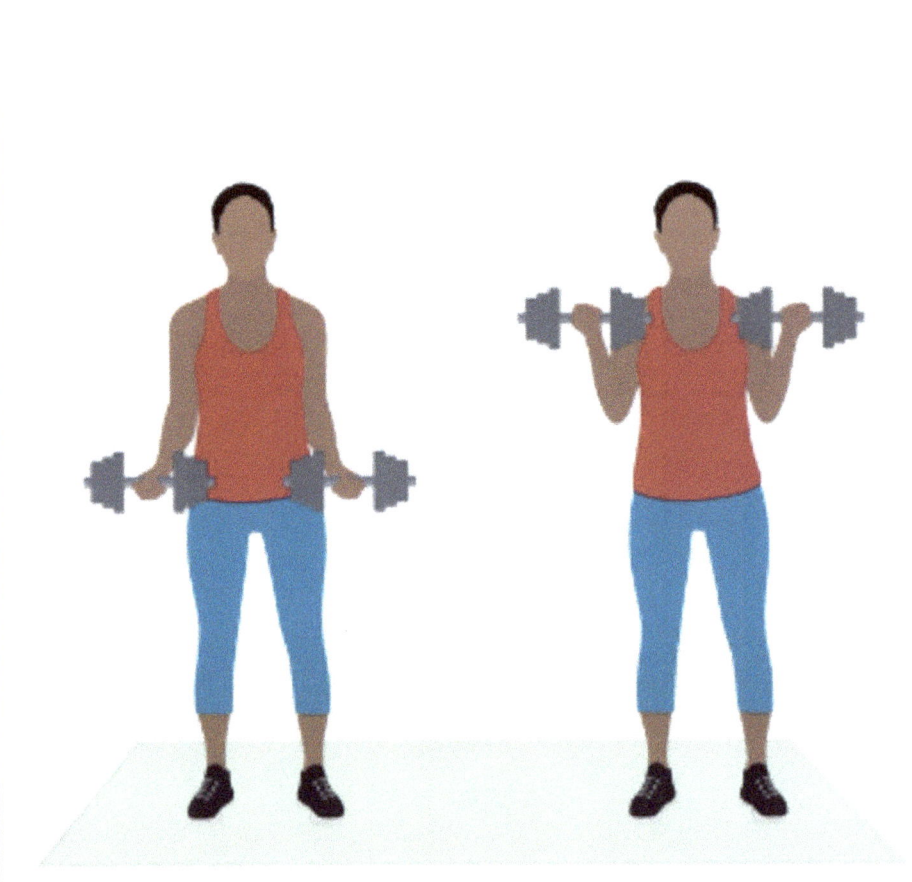

Dumbbell Bicep Curls

Stand with feet shoulder width apart, hold dumbbells at arm's length, then curl them towards your shoulders.

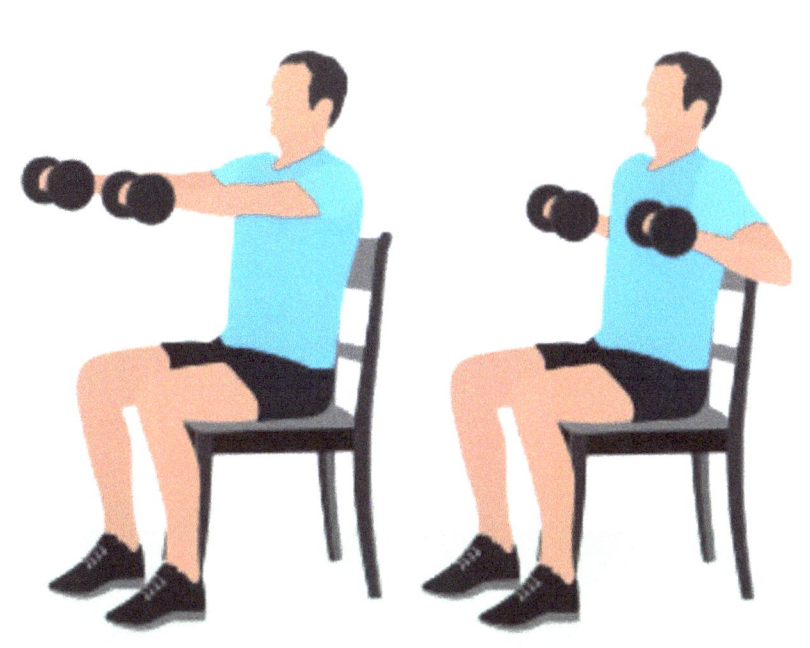

Dumbbell Chest Press

Sit on the chair, hold a dumbbell in each hand at chest level, and press them forward until your arms are fully extended, maintaining the horizontal position.

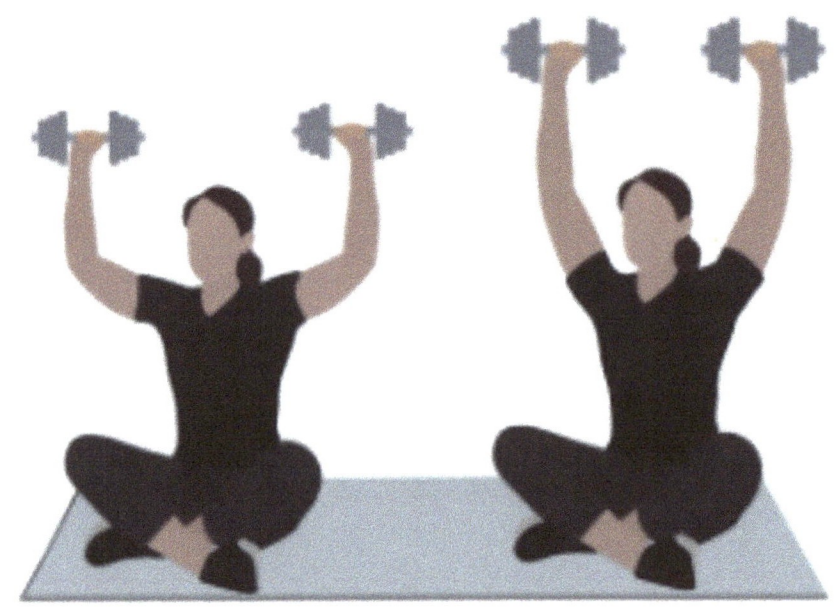

Dumbbell Shoulder Press in Indian Seats

Sit cross-legged on a mat, holding dumbbells at shoulder height, then press them upward and lower them back down while seated.

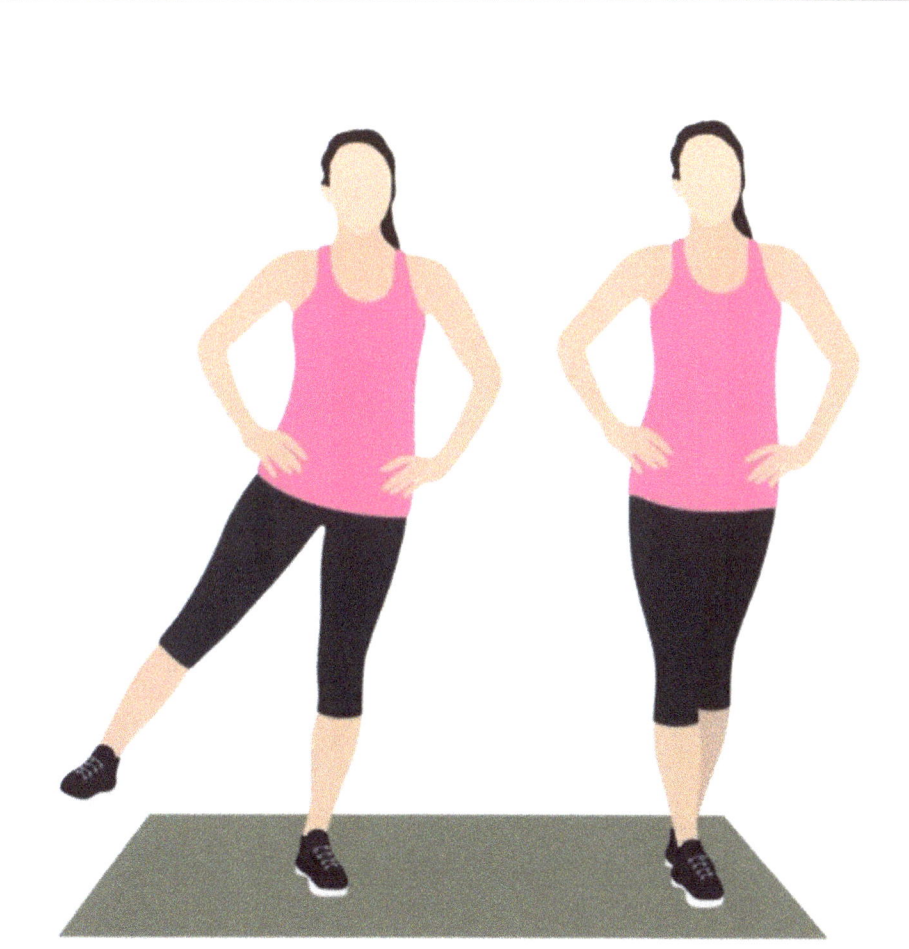

Lateral Leg Raises

Stand on one leg, lift the other leg out to the side, then lower it back down, alternate legs.

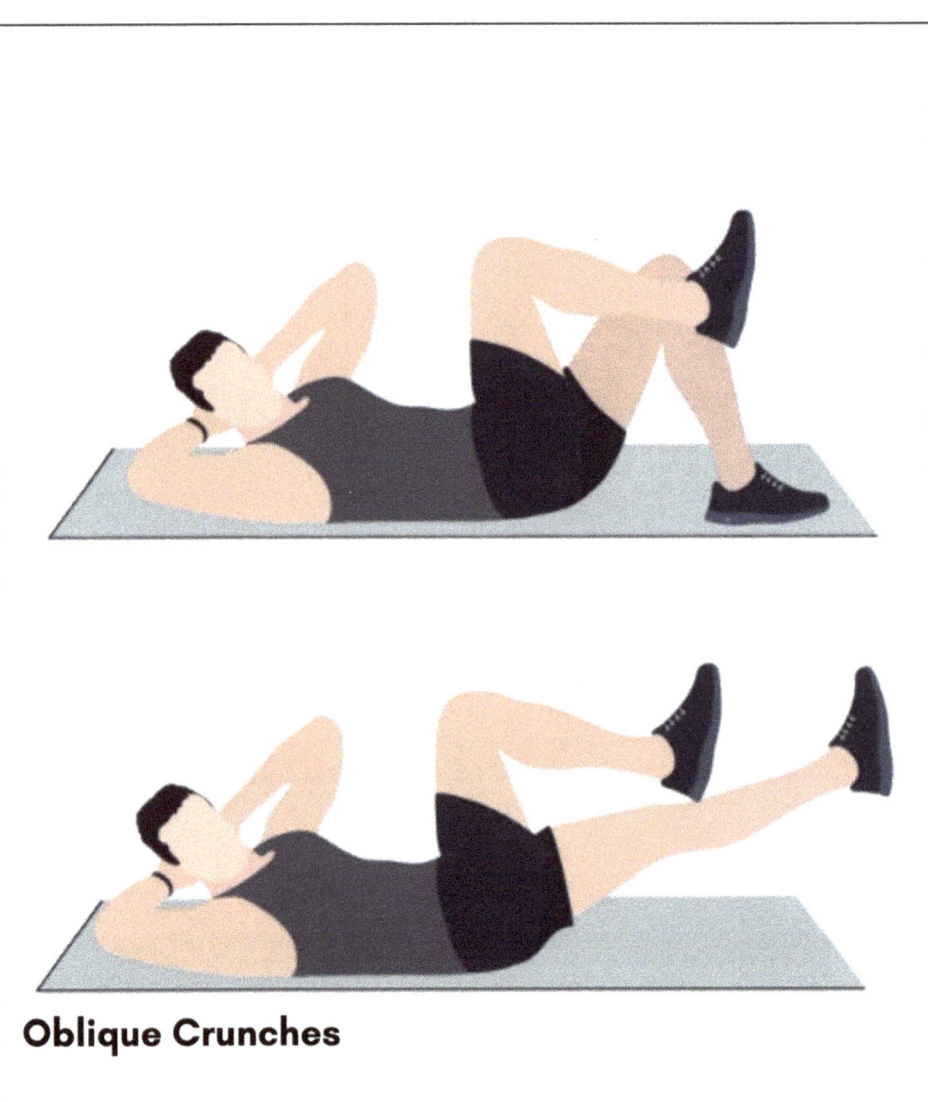

Oblique Crunches

Lie on your back, knees bent, and perform a crunch by bringing your elbow towards the opposite knee, engaging the oblique muscles on each side.

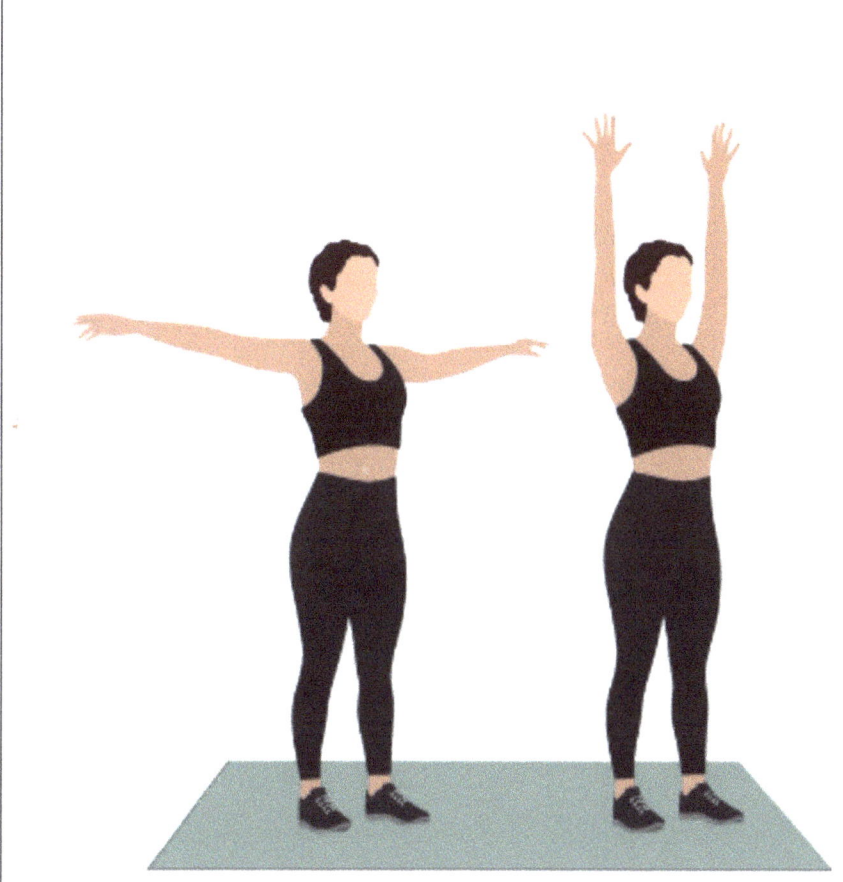

Overhead Lateral Raise

From a standing position, raise both arms out to the sides and overhead, then lower them back down to shoulder level.

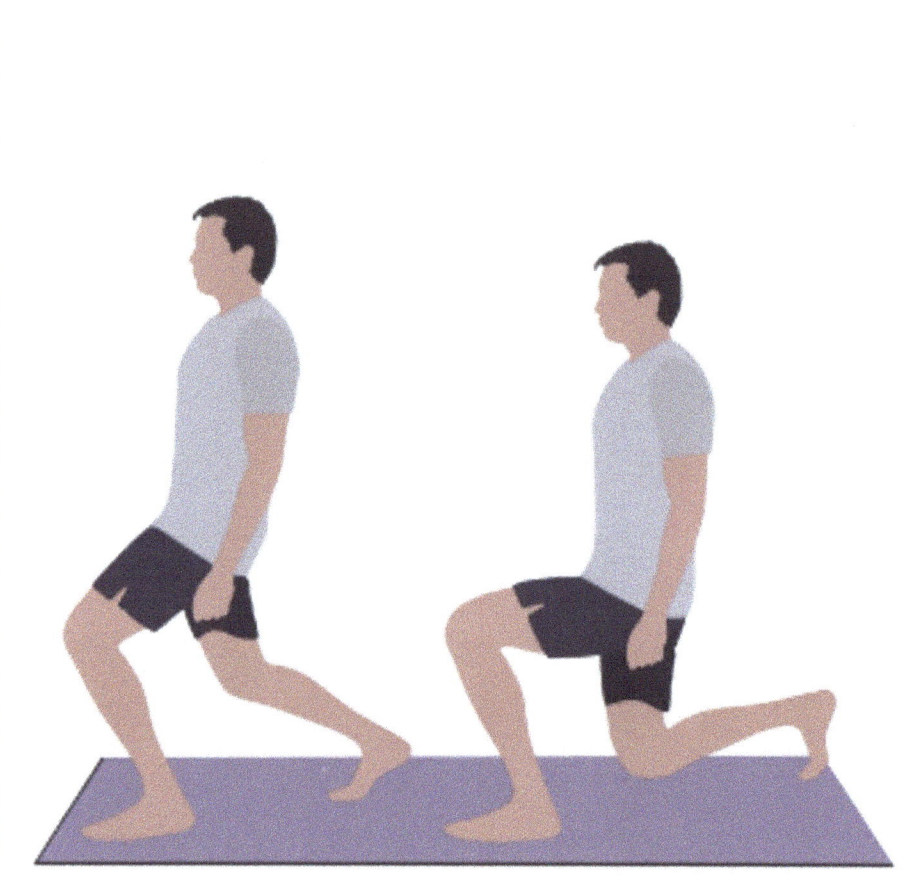

Pulse Lunges

Perform a regular lunge, but instead of returning to the starting position, pulse up and down slightly before standing up.

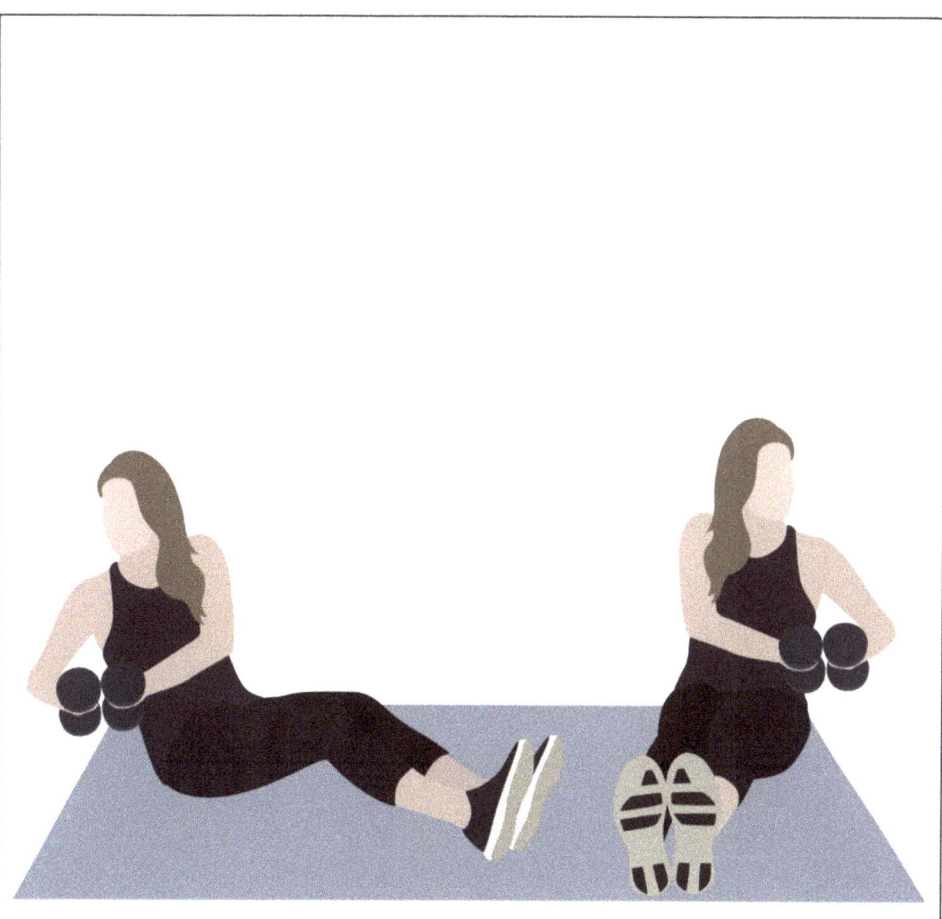

Russian Twist with Dumbbell

Sit on a mat, lift feet, hold a dumbbell, and twist your torso, touching the dumbbell near each hip alternately.

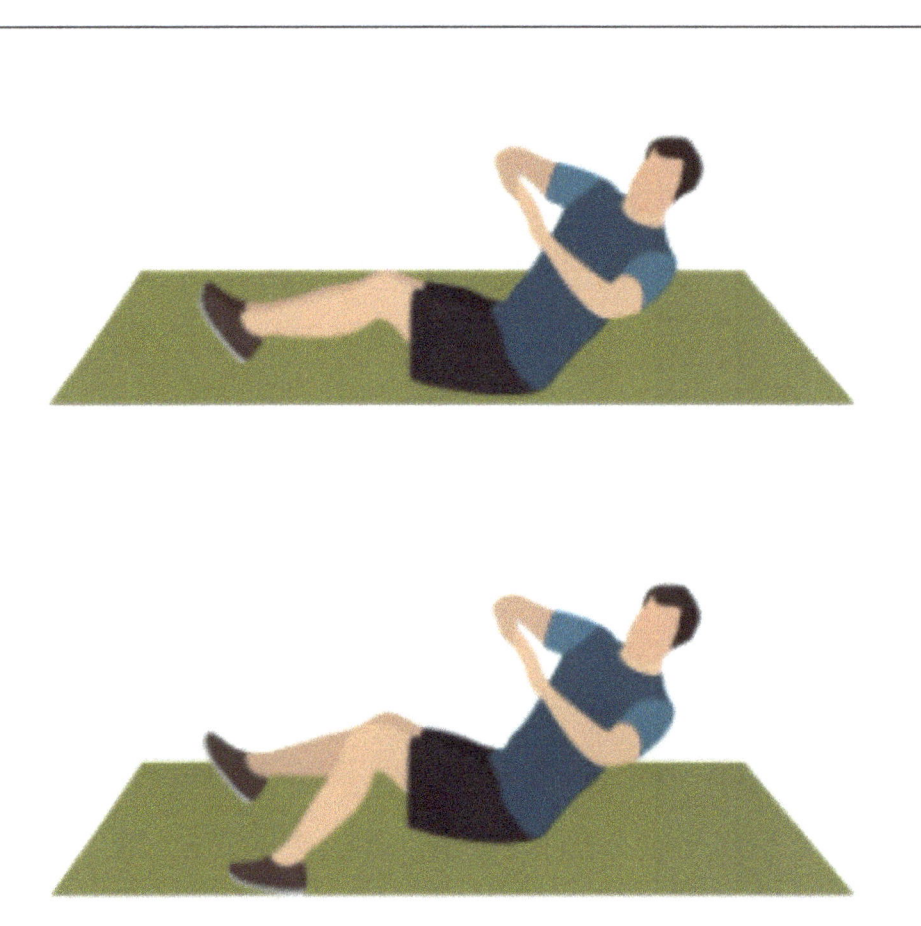

Russian Twists

Lie on your back, lift your upper body, and twist your torso to each side, touching the floor beside you.

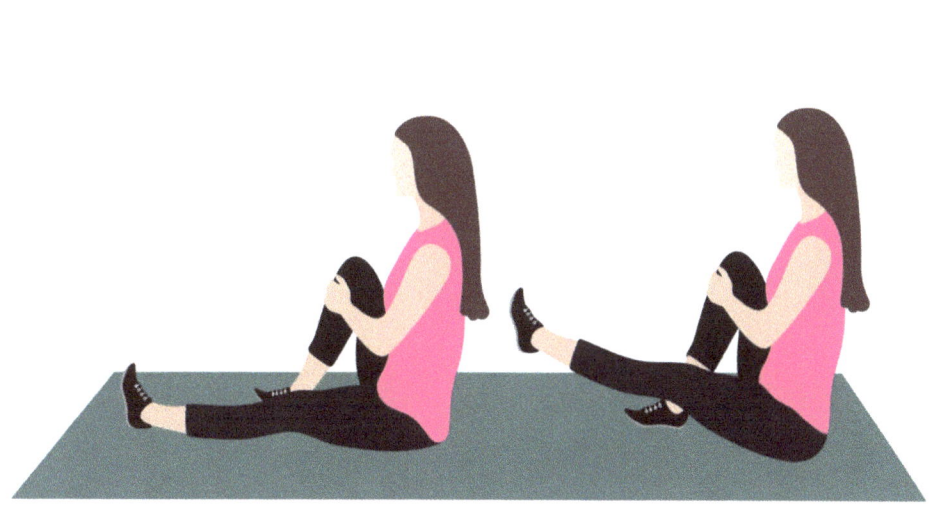

Seated Straight Leg Raise with Bent Knee

Sit with one knee bent and one leg straight.
Lift the straight leg while engaging your core.
Alternate between legs.

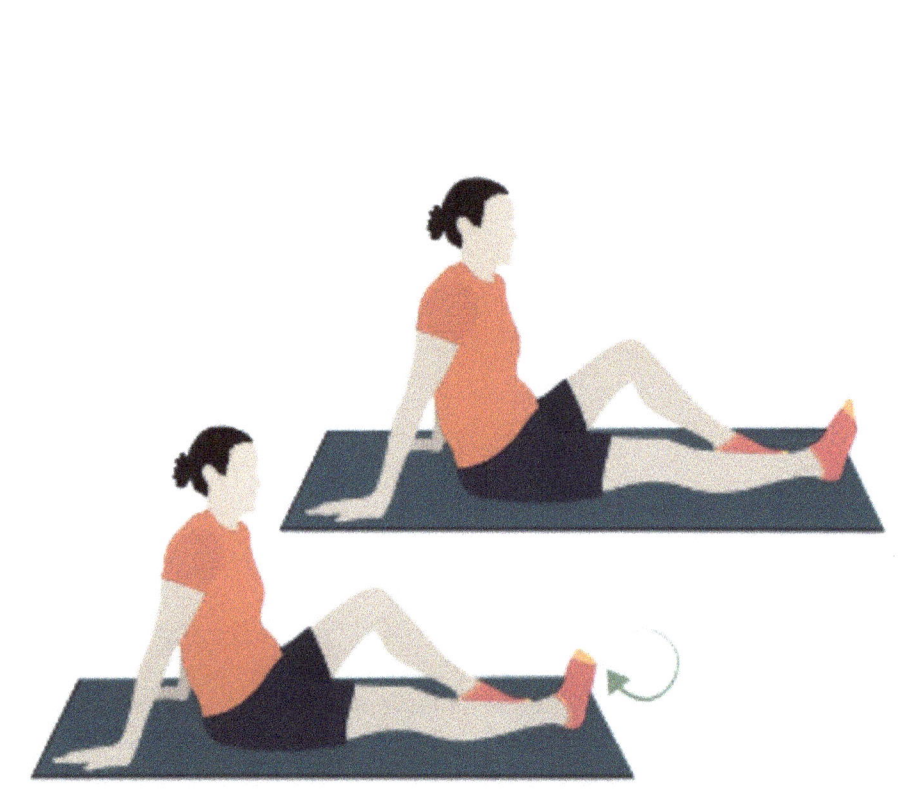

Seated Straight Leg Raises

Sit on the mat with your legs extended straight out in front of you. Lift one leg at a time straight up off the mat, keeping your knees straight and engaging your core. Alternate between legs.

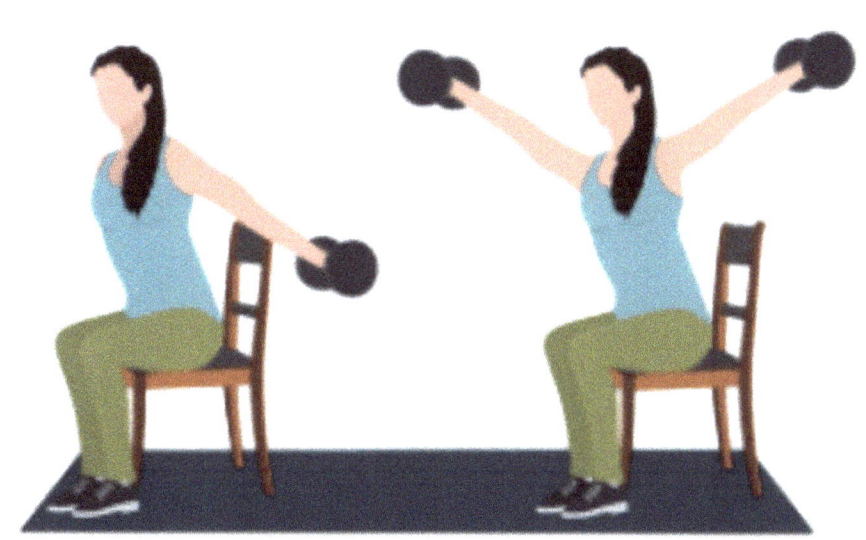

Seated Y Raises

Sit on the chair, lean forward slightly, arms extended in a Y shape, lift them up to shoulder height, then lower them back down.

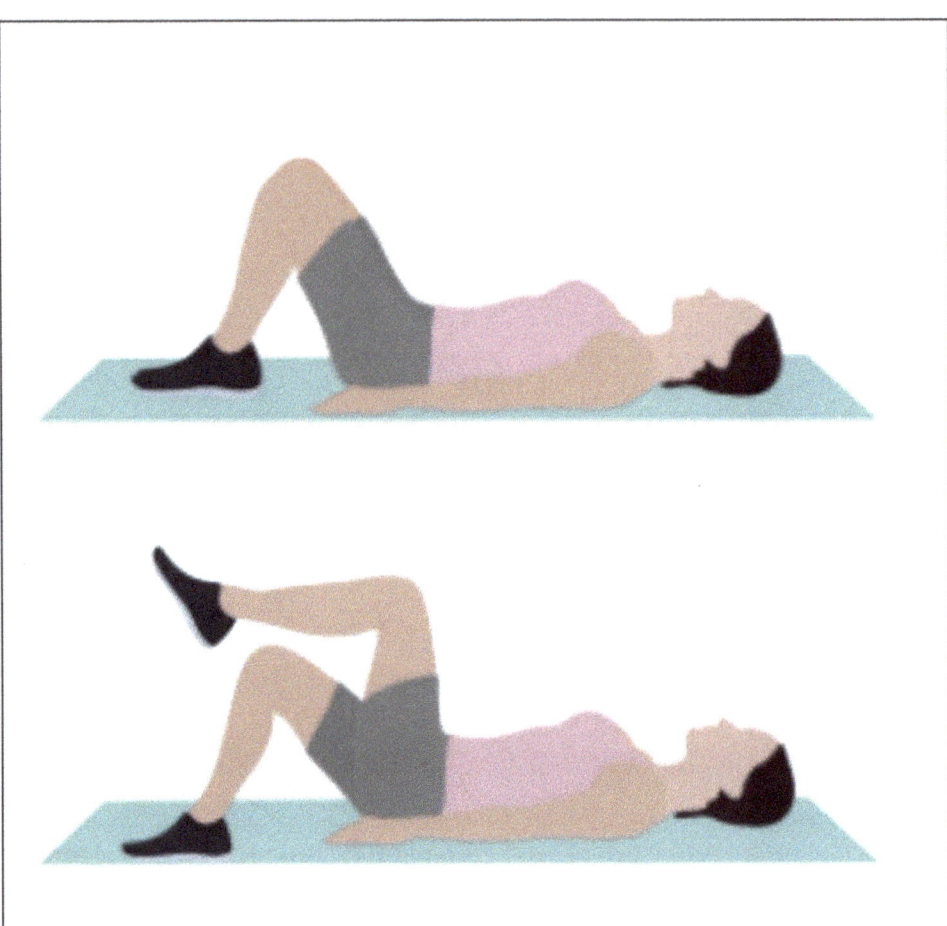

Single Leg Bent Knee Leg Raises

Lie on your back, knees bent, and lift your legs towards the ceiling while keeping them bent.

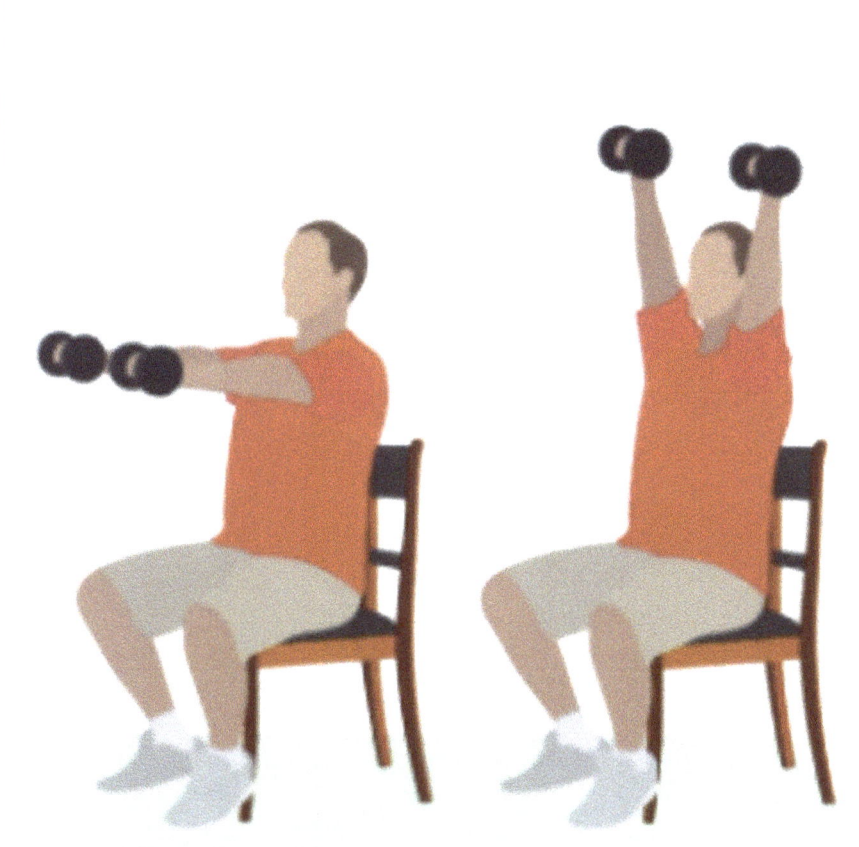

Seated Dumbbell Front Raises

Sit on a chair, hold a dumbbell in each hand, arms extended straight down in front of you, raise both arms forward and upward to shoulder level, then lower them back down.

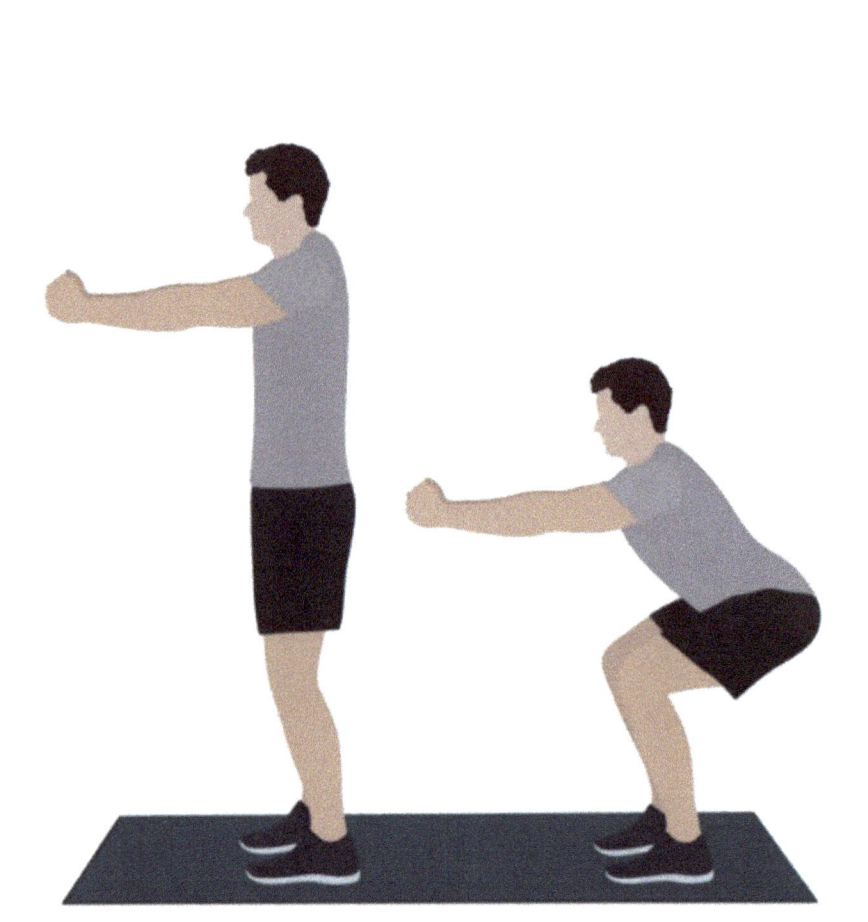

Squat with Lateral Hand Raise

Squat down, then as you rise, extend both arms out to the sides at shoulder level, and lower them as you squat again.

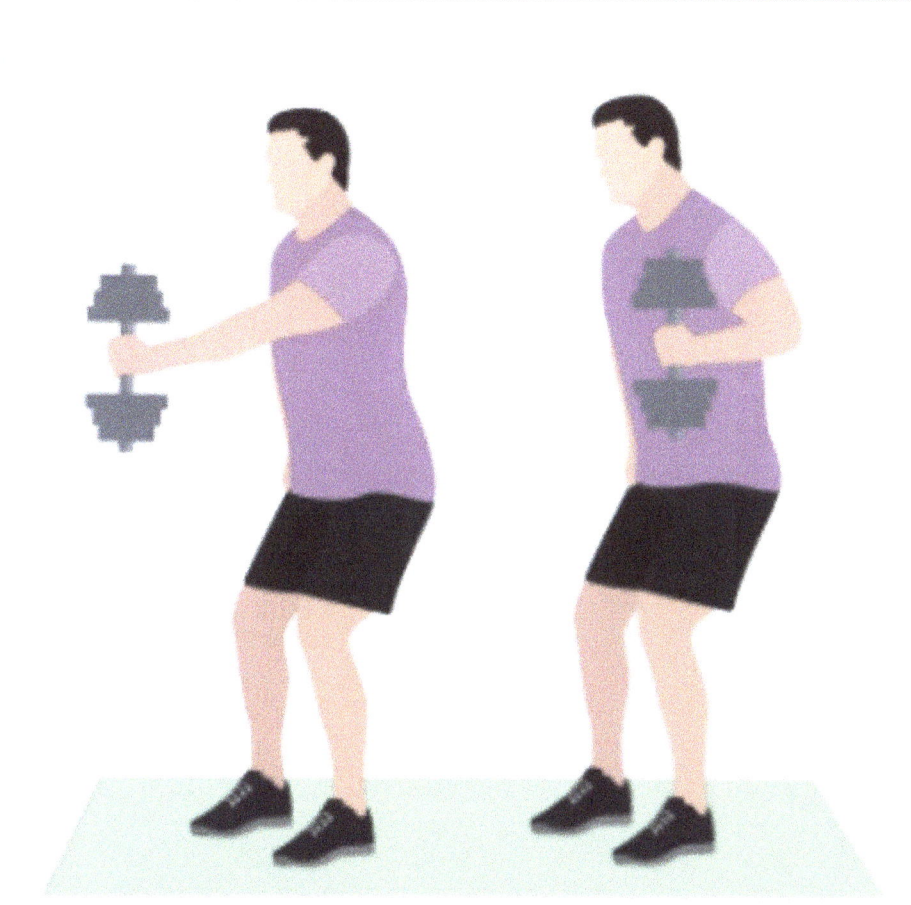

Standing Bent Over Dumbbell Row

Hinge at hips, keep back flat, hold dumbbells, pull towards chest, elbows close, shoulder blades squeezed, return to start.

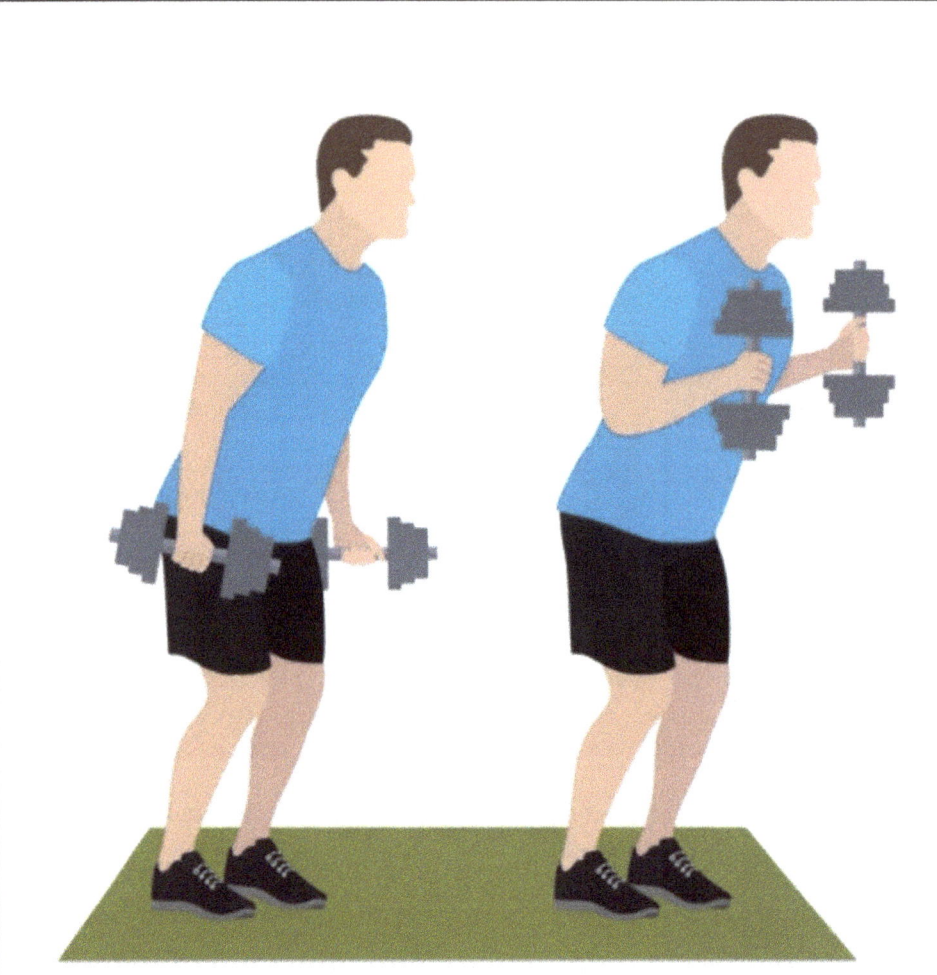

Standing Dumbbell Hammer Curls

Stand with feet shoulder-width apart, hold dumbbells with palms facing inward, then curl them towards your shoulders.

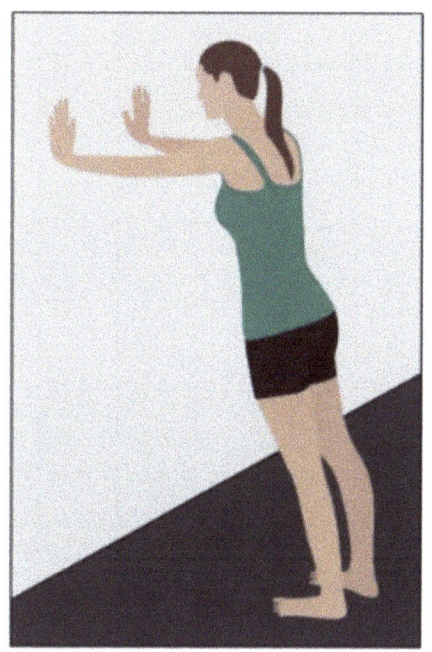 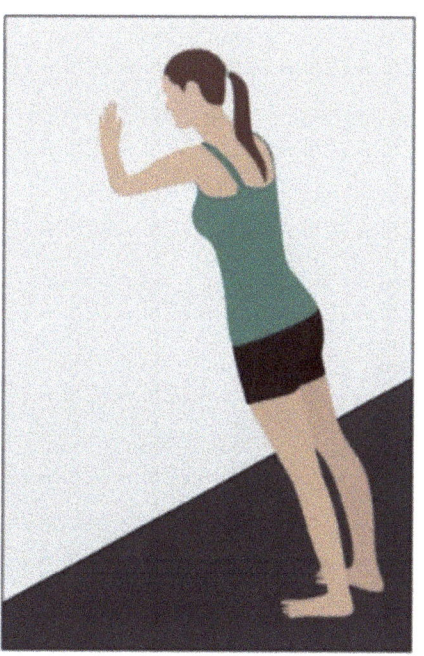

Wall Push-Up

Stand facing a wall, place hands on the wall at shoulder height, and push away from the wall.

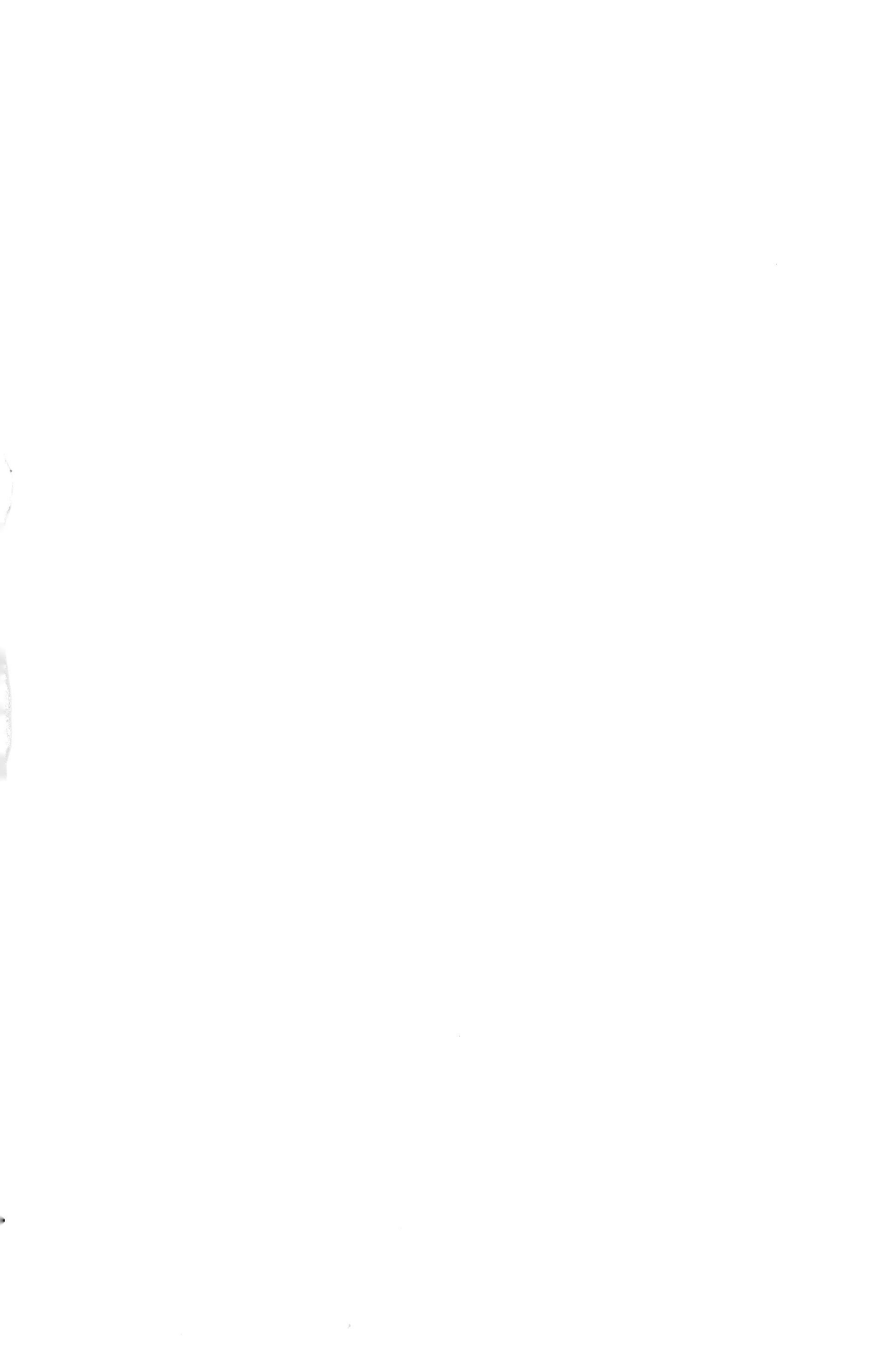

www.ingramcontent.com/pod-product-compliance
Lightning Source LLC
Chambersburg PA
CBHW040222040426
42333CB00051B/3300